Mindfulness Journal for Depression

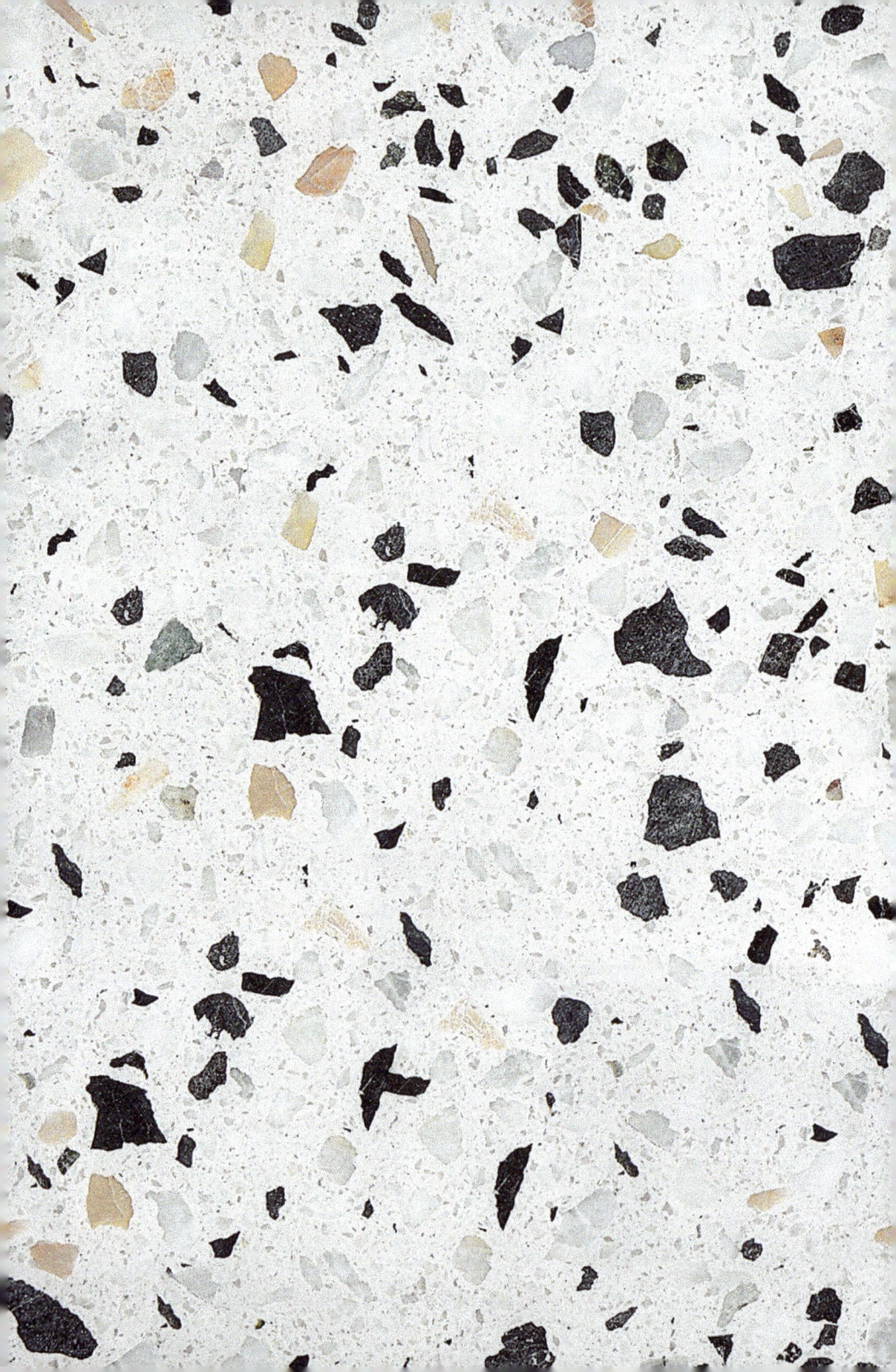

Mindfulness Journal
for Depression

A Guided Journey Toward Self-Compassion and Positivity

TANYA J. PETERSON

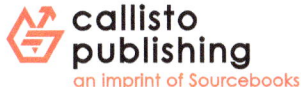
an imprint of Sourcebooks

Copyright © 2021 by Callisto Publishing LLC
Cover and internal design © 2021 by Callisto Publishing LLC
Illustrations © Basia Stryjecka/Creative Market; Lisima/Creative Market; Trezvo/Shutterstock
Author photo courtesy of Shanna Chess
Interior and Cover Designer: Jennifer Hsu
Art Producer: Meg Baggott
Editor: Jesse Aylen
Production Editor: Ruth Sakata Corley
Production Manager: Holly Haydash

Callisto and the colophon are registered trademarks of Callisto Publishing LLC.

All rights reserved. No part of this book may be reproduced in any form or by any electronic or mechanical means including information storage and retrieval systems—except in the case of brief quotations embodied in critical articles or reviews—without permission in writing from its publisher, Sourcebooks LLC.

All brand names and product names used in this book are trademarks, registered trademarks, or trade names of their respective holders. Callisto Publishing is not associated with any product or vendor in this book.

This book is not intended as a substitute for medical advice from a qualified physician. The intent of this book is to provide accurate general information in regard to the subject matter covered. If medical advice or other expert help is needed, the services of an appropriate medical professional should be sought.

Published by Callisto Publishing LLC C/O Sourcebooks LLC
P.O. Box 4410, Naperville, Illinois 60567-4410
(630) 961-3900
callistopublishing.com

Printed in the United States of America.

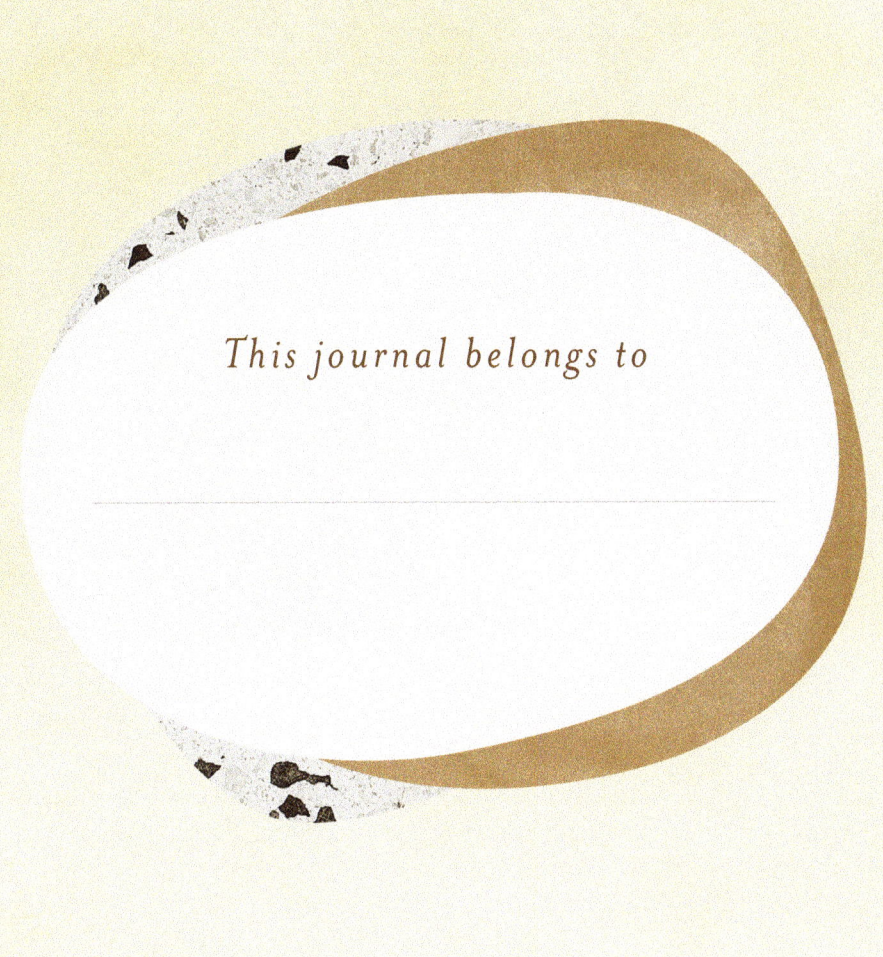

This journal belongs to

_____

"IF YOU ARE ALWAYS TRYING TO BE NORMAL, YOU WILL NEVER KNOW HOW AMAZING YOU CAN BE."

—*Maya Angelou*

CONTENTS

INTRODUCTION *viii*

HOW TO USE THIS JOURNAL *x*

    Thoughts Are Not Facts *1*

    Notice, But Don't Dwell *45*

    Depression Doesn't Define Me *87*

    The Mindful Way *129*

RESOURCES *172*

REFERENCES *175*

INTRODUCTION

WELCOME TO THIS JOURNAL, THIS EXPERIENCE—and this moment. Embrace the fact that you are on this journey to well-being, a process of breaking free from your mind to live fully in each moment of your life, through all its ups and downs. Be grateful to yourself for picking up this journal and diving in, for doing this is no small act. Many people *want* to change their relationship with themselves, their challenges, or life itself, and you are actually *doing* it. That takes courage and strength, so own it and be proud!

It's especially important to appreciate yourself and acknowledge any positive action you take when you're experiencing depression, general low mood, lack of motivation, burnout, or are simply not feeling the way you want to feel. Negative thoughts and feelings can be overwhelming and overpowering, affecting you completely and interfering in your life. Perhaps you picked up this journal because you want to understand yourself better. Maybe you'd like to explore challenging situations or specific people, events, and experiences that trigger negative thoughts and emotions. Quite possibly, you're interested in developing a new way of being, thinking, feeling, and doing. I'd venture to guess that you are tired of living under the weight of depression or negativity. To that end, know that you are in the right place at the right time: here, with this journal, in this moment. You're about to engage, learn, discover, and grow.

I come to you from both a professional and a personal background in mental health struggles—and soaring past them in a new way by living mindfully. I've been a teacher and a counselor, and now I've turned to writing so I can help people find and use practical tools to shape the person they want to be and create the life they want to live. Personally, I've lived with anxiety for much of my life. I sustained a traumatic brain injury in a car accident and two smaller concussions shortly after, and I experienced a period of such emotional upheaval that I was diagnosed with bipolar disorder. I've since discovered a new way of being with myself and my life, and I created this journal because I know what it's like both to experience difficulty and to transcend it. I offer this journal to you for your own journey to well-being.

You'll explore yourself and learn how to embrace mindful living using evidence-based prompts and techniques so you can live fully, no longer held back by negative thoughts, low mood, and lack of energy. This journal is based on mindfulness-based cognitive therapy (MBCT), a well-researched approach to wellness that was originally created to help people prevent depression relapse by expanding their relationship with the thoughts and feelings of depression. MBCT practices are designed to help you move away from being stuck in depressive thoughts to a place where you can directly experience these thoughts in new and helpful ways. MBCT itself is a structured, 8-week group program. This journal draws on the basic principles of it. The "mindfulness" component is about developing a new presence with yourself and in your life, and the "cognitive" aspect helps you understand and become more aware of negative thoughts that are getting in your way.

The breathing exercises, body scans, meditations, movement exercises, and mindfulness techniques of MBCT can help you break out of the cycle of depression. Automatic negative thoughts are a hallmark of depression. They are habitual patterns of thinking that cause us to negatively interpret situations, other people, and even ourselves. They're not something you do on purpose. The human brain looks for problems so it can fix them, and sometimes our thoughts get stuck in negativity. These negative thoughts directly influence your mood and emotions, and thoughts, moods, and emotions directly influence your actions. Actions, in turn, further influence thoughts and emotions, and it's easy to become caught up in a negative loop.

By developing awareness of yourself, your thoughts, and the moments of your life, you can experience life fully—and thrive.

HOW TO USE THIS JOURNAL

This is *your* journal. You and your depression are unique. Therefore, instead of dictating rules for using your own journal on your journey to a new relationship with yourself, I offer you some suggestions to maximize your experience.

This journal is structured in four parts. In the first part, you'll discover why you can't always believe your thoughts. Next, you'll learn how to notice your thoughts and feelings without becoming stuck in them. Then, you'll explore the depths of who you are—and begin to see that you are most definitely not your depression. Finally, you'll begin to cultivate a new way of being, embracing the mindful way of life for deep well-being. Although each part can stand alone, I suggest that you work through the journal in order, because with each part, you'll gain new awareness that will carry into the next.

Above all, be patient and gentle with yourself. Depression is persistent and doesn't just disappear. It will throw obstacles in your way. You might find it difficult to concentrate at times, with your mind distracted and wandering to problems and doubts; you might forget to journal sometimes or feel guilty taking this time for yourself; you might notice discomfort and want to avoid it. Know that these are common roadblocks along the journey to freedom and well-being. Making journaling a routine can help overcome these roadblocks. Try to journal regularly (perhaps daily or three times per week). Enjoy your journal mindfully. This simply means paying attention fully whenever you journal and noticing how you feel during your experience. Also, creating a ritual around journaling—such as sitting in a favorite spot with a special pen, a candle, and a cup of hot tea—will help you look forward to this valuable time.

    Finally, set your own pace. Don't rush yourself or see this as something to push through so you can finally feel better. This isn't a quick-fix manual, but a process of discovery and becoming. You might find it helpful to use it in conjunction with other treatment for depression, such as medication or therapy, as this isn't intended to be a replacement for those helpful methodologies. Your commitment to journaling is powerful and can help get you where you want to be. Depression isn't who you are, and moods don't define you! You have within you the strength and ability to break free from it, and you've already begun your journey to the quality life you want to live—on your terms. My sincere hope is that you enjoy this process of taking back your life.

Thoughts Are Not Facts

Thoughts are ideas formed in your mind. They're not concrete, hard-and-fast, tangible truths. But they seem believable because they come from your mind. You wouldn't lie to yourself, would you? Actually, you likely often do, as it's simply what the human brain does—looking for problems so you're aware of things that could go wrong. Therefore, in most cases, you don't purposefully deceive yourself; you think you're telling yourself truthful things.

Researchers have discovered that about 70 percent of your thoughts are negative and that you're often not fully aware of them. They come automatically, as an undercurrent of negativity clouding your perception and causing you to impose judgment on yourself, others, and situations around you. They're always in the background and can feel uncontrollable, popping up when you least expect them. Negative thoughts, emotions, and actions taken (or not taken) can feed on each other and spiral, leading to a sense of despair, loss, hopelessness, listlessness, burnout, self-criticism, resentment, guilt, or anger. That is depression: exhausting, all-consuming, making it difficult to concentrate on anything else. But when you become aware of those negative thoughts, you gain the upper hand.

Mindfulness can help, bringing your thoughts and emotions into your awareness. As you work through this part of your journal, you'll boost your mindfulness skills, increasing awareness around your negative thoughts and coming to a clearer understanding of your depression or low mood and lack of energy.

WHAT EXPERIENCES, THOUGHTS, and feelings prompted you to pick up this journal? Describe them here to bring them into your full awareness.

WHEN ARE YOU most aware of these experiences, thoughts, and feelings? At first, it might seem like your emotions, thoughts, and energy levels are always the same. However, it's likely that they do change, but it's so subtle that you don't notice shifts. Begin to notice when you feel better and when you feel worse and note it here.

WHAT IS HAPPENING when your thoughts are most negative and you feel the lowest? (Notice time of day, situations, levels of hunger or thirst, etc.)

WHAT IS HAPPENING when your thoughts are more neutral, or even positive, and you feel better?

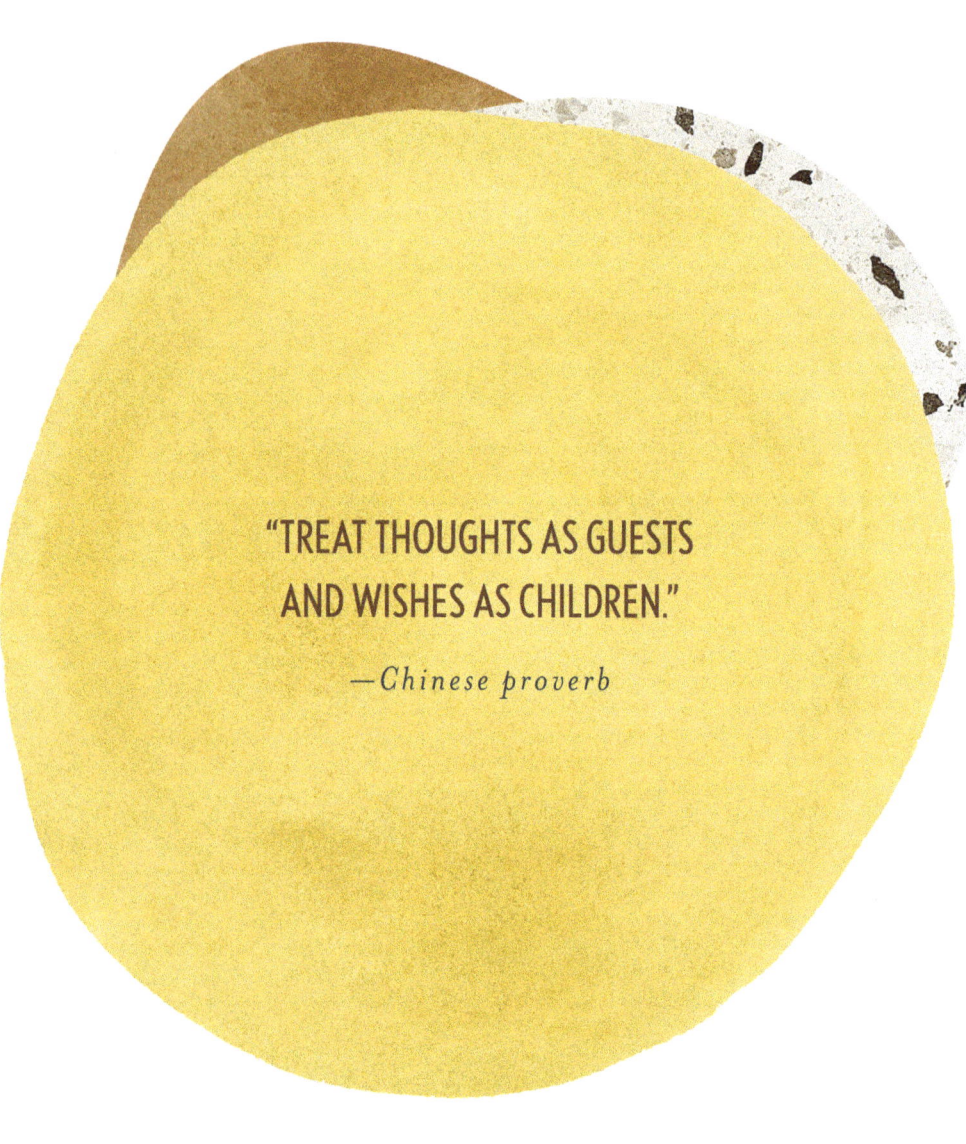

"TREAT THOUGHTS AS GUESTS
AND WISHES AS CHILDREN."

—*Chinese proverb*

BUDDY UP TO YOUR BREATH

Your breath is one of those automatic body functions that your brain and nervous system handle. You don't have to think about breathing or try to remember to breathe. Therefore, most of us don't pay a bit of attention to the act and experience of breathing. However, the breath is actually a powerful ally that gives you access to your inner workings. By breathing slowly and deeply, you can turn off your sympathetic nervous system (that causes your stress reaction) and instead activate the parasympathetic nervous system (that calms you down).

The first step in using your breath to impact your mood and experience is to understand that it's a friend you can play with to bring mental health benefits. Therefore, this very first breath exercise is just about observing. Don't try to change anything. Simply become aware of your breathing.

- Notice your body in whatever position you are in, whether you're standing, sitting, or lying down.
- Become aware that you are breathing. Notice the sound and feel of your breath as it enters and leaves your body.
- As you inhale, say to yourself, "Hello, breath," just as if you are greeting a friend.
- As you exhale, say to yourself, "Goodbye, breath," as if you are departing from a friend.
- Do this several times each day. Start with just 30 seconds at a time, and when your mind wanders, simply return your attention to your breath.

HOW CAN BEING aware of your unique patterns of thinking and feeling make a difference in your emotional state? What actions might you take to put you in charge of your ups and downs so you don't feel at the mercy of your moods?

WHAT ARE YOU thinking right now? Chances are, you'll start to notice a flood of thoughts. Don't try to change them. Simply jot down all thoughts that come to mind in the next three to five minutes.

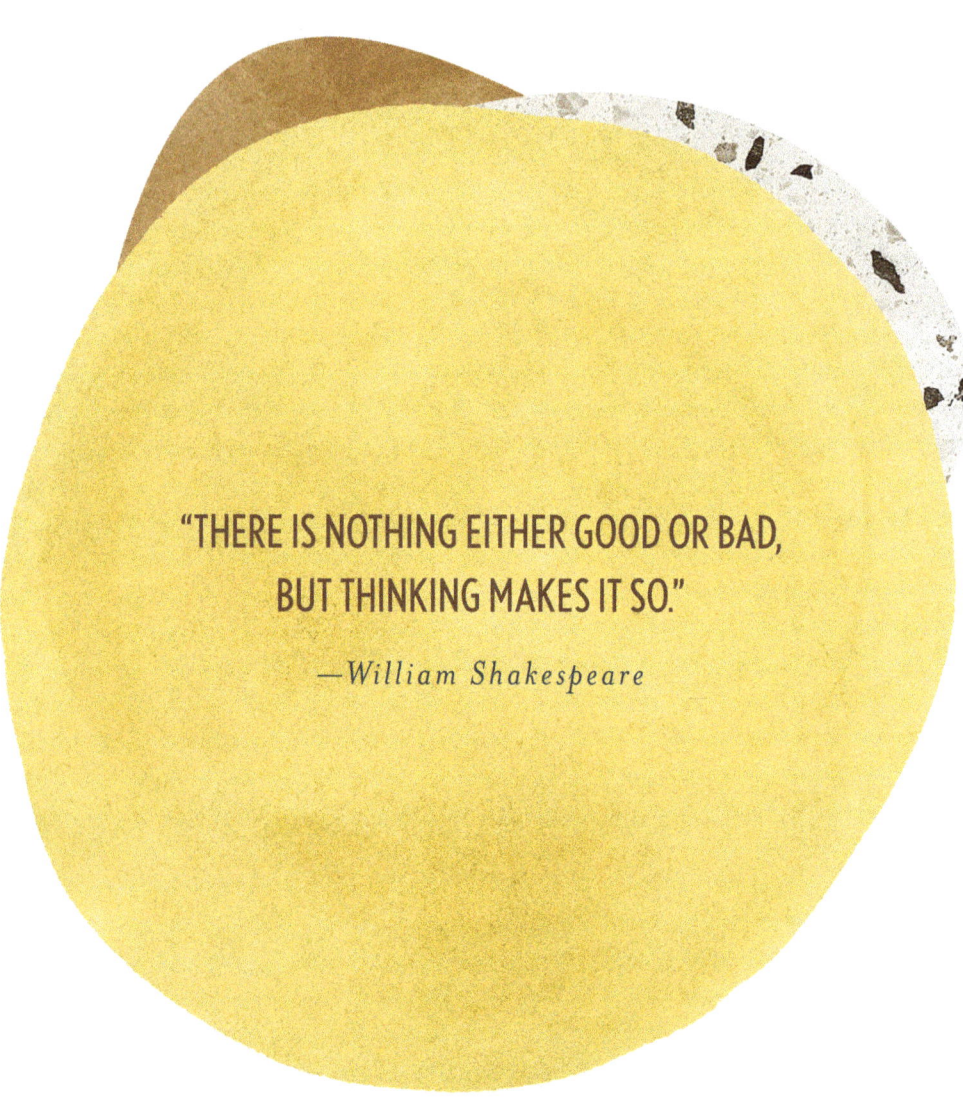

"THERE IS NOTHING EITHER GOOD OR BAD,
BUT THINKING MAKES IT SO."

—*William Shakespeare*

HOW DID WRITING down your thoughts impact your emotions? List the feelings that emerged when you wrote down your thoughts.

THOUGHTS OFTEN RUN in the background. You're not fully aware of them, yet you're affected by them. Consider your list of thoughts on page 9. Using these or adding to them, make a "top thoughts" list of 10 of your most bothersome negative thoughts.

NOW THAT THEY'RE out of your unconscious mind and onto paper in front of you, consider your top negative thoughts. Don't judge yourself for having these thoughts! Remember that they're automatic and you're not intentionally thinking them. Noticing and exploring them without being hard on yourself can help you free yourself. Being completely honest with yourself, how accurate are they? Give examples of times when these thoughts aren't true.

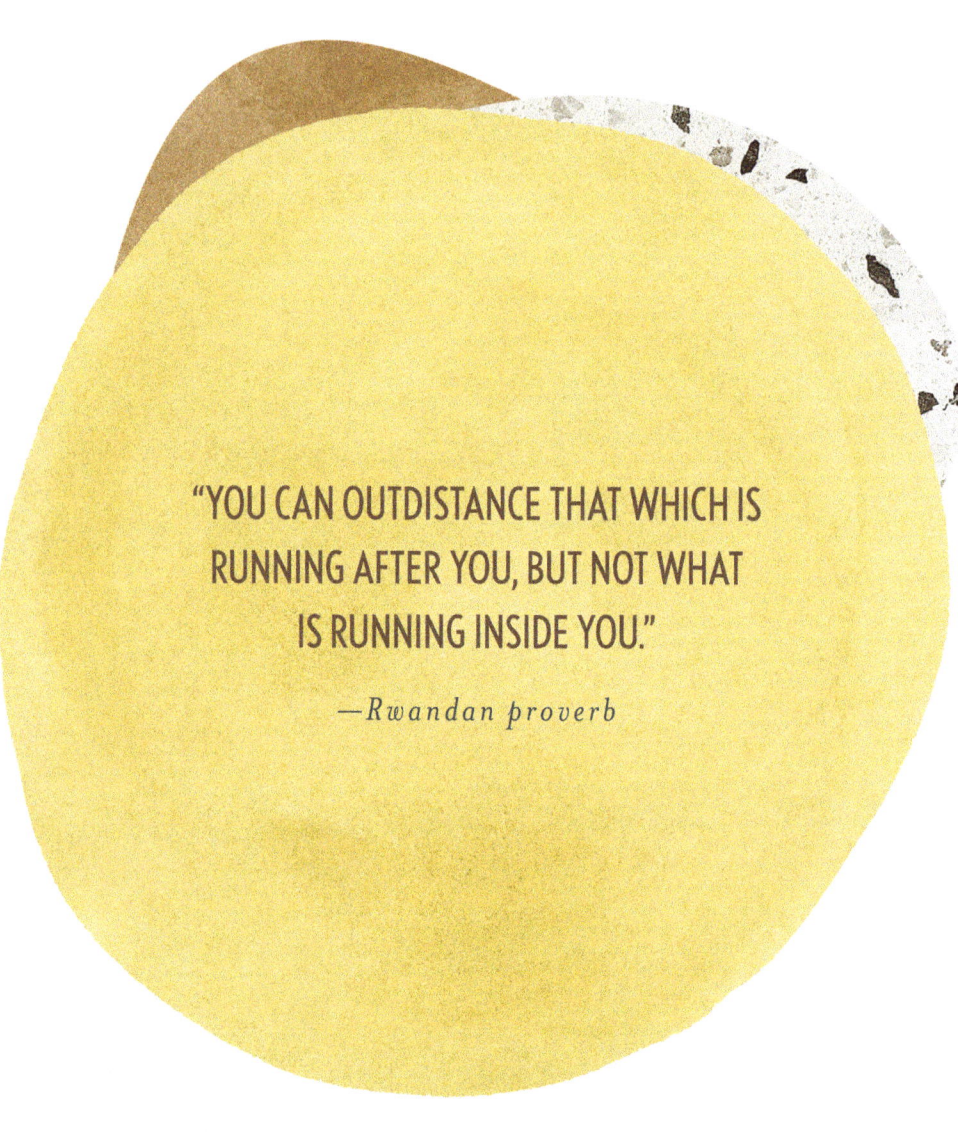

"YOU CAN OUTDISTANCE THAT WHICH IS RUNNING AFTER YOU, BUT NOT WHAT IS RUNNING INSIDE YOU."

—*Rwandan proverb*

WHERE DO YOUR THOUGHTS SHOW UP IN YOUR BODY?

The mind and body aren't two distinct components independent of each other. Your thoughts don't just stay in your head. They reverberate through your entire being and can cause aches, pains, and tension. Take a moment to examine where they show up:

- Sit or lie comfortably.
- Close your eyes and turn your attention to your body. Notice how you feel.
- Call to mind one of the negative thoughts that often pops into your head. Pay attention to the thought.
- Now, turn your attention to your body again, tuning in to each distinct part. What do you notice now?
- Write down any physical sensations that appeared or intensified when you were thinking about your negative thought.

_____

_____

_____

_____

_____

_____

THINK OF A recent situation that was difficult for you. If you feel comfortable doing so, I invite you to imagine that it is happening again right now. What is going on? What thoughts, emotions, and physical sensations are you experiencing?

REMEMBERING AN EXPERIENCE is often different from the initial experience. Were you as aware of your thoughts and feelings when you were actively experiencing that difficult situation? What is different about remembering it versus experiencing it? Is it the same?

BEING STUCK IN thoughts about what has already happened can keep negative thoughts and emotions alive, but it also gives you a chance to look at the situation differently. Write down one or two thoughts you have about the experience from page 16.

Now that there's some distance between you and your initial thoughts about the situation, write down new interpretations of your initial reaction.

GO DEEPER WITH this, and look back to the prompt on page 8 where you reflected on how being aware of your unique thinking patterns makes a difference in your emotional state. What new actions can you add to the list you made? What new things can you do based on your new interpretations?

GROUND YOURSELF WITH A FOCUS OBJECT

Focus objects are useful mindfulness tools that provide something tangible to divert your attention from your inner ruminations. A focus object is anything you want it to be and is merely something in your immediate vicinity that you can notice with your senses.

Your thoughts and feelings are experienced in your mind. Separate yourself from them by purposefully paying attention to what you are doing in the present moment. Place your attention on one single thing. This might be an object, a person, or a sound. Notice it fully and completely. Note as many details about your focus object as you can, mentally describing the nuances of what you see, hear, feel, and/or smell. Don't judge it; just observe it. When other thoughts or evaluations creep in, return your concentration to the object in this moment.

OFTEN, WE SEE our thoughts in new ways when we look at them from different perspectives. From that top 10 list of bothersome negative thoughts you generated on page 12, select one and describe a situation in which this thought was strong.

NOW, IMAGINE YOU are watching this scenario from above, as if you are a bird who has no connection to the situation you're watching. Describe how you see it from this neutral position.

NOW VISUALIZE THIS situation from the perspective of a trusted friend or loved one. What do they see?

HOW DO THESE two new perspectives (as a distant observer from above and as someone who cares about you) influence your original interpretation? How do they influence your negative thought and the emotions connected to it?

PRACTICE BEING A NEUTRAL OBSERVER

The negative thoughts and feelings of depression have a way of imposing themselves on your sense of self and most situations in your life. As humans, we have a natural tendency to judge ourselves, others, and situations as "good" or "bad." But your thoughts about things aren't always accurate, nor do they define what something is really like. The truth is that things simply exist. Situations are what they are. When you drop judgment, you have a chance to respond differently. Today, practice simply noticing yourself and aspects of your life as a neutral observer; someone who has no emotional connection to what is on your radar. Practice looking around you and describing what you see in objective terms.

HOW DO YOU tend to react to your negative thoughts and feelings? Think of actions you take, actions you don't take, impulses you have, etc.

HOW DO YOU tend to respond to your positive thoughts and feelings?

WHAT IS HAPPENING differently when you have negative thoughts compared to positive thoughts? How does the quality of your thoughts influence your feelings and actions?

THOUGHTS HAVE A way of popping into your mind in quick succession, one leading to another and then another. They behave much like popcorn kernels as they begin to heat up and burst open. The difference is that popcorn is loud, and you know what's happening when it's popping. Thoughts are sneakier and more insidious, and they can explode out of control before you realize it. Write down one negative thought that often pops into your head.

DEVELOP MINDFUL AWARENESS OF WHAT'S INFLUENCING YOUR THOUGHTS AND MOOD

Begin to actively notice your thoughts and mood. Rather than trying to force a shift in how you feel, become aware of what is going on in the moment. Observe yourself and your surroundings. What do you need right now? Do you need a glass of water? Something nutritious to eat? Some movement to get your energy flowing? A bit of quiet to reduce stimulation? Practice being aware of the situation underlying your mood so you can take one small action to feel better.

WHAT OTHER THOUGHTS, feelings, or memories does the negative thought you wrote on page 29 automatically spark? Write down everything that comes to mind in the chain reaction.

WHAT DO YOU notice about the kernels of thought that exploded? Do you notice any patterns? How would you summarize the theme of your thoughts? (For example, you might notice themes of guilt, worthlessness, disappointment, or negative interpretations of people and situations.)

ANALYZING YOUR THOUGHT patterns may be uncomfortable, but know that it has a purpose. It helps you develop deeper awareness, and it is only through awareness of your experiences that you can fully embrace yourself and transform in meaningful ways. Ponder the chain reaction of your thoughts further. Imagine they were all absolutely true. How does this affect your emotions? Sensations in your body? What does it make you want to do or not do?

CONSIDER THE INITIAL negative thought you wrote about on page 29 more neutrally, like an investigator who knows nothing about a case and is searching for facts. What evidence does the investigator find that proves the thought is true? What evidence does the investigator find that proves the thought isn't true?

FROM AN MBCT-BASED perspective, events are neutral. Your thoughts about an event impact how you feel and the actions you take. Practice separating your thoughts about a circumstance from the situation itself. Start by selecting another one of your top negative thoughts from page 12 (pick a new one) and writing down a recent time it was in your mind.

PAUSE AND SIMPLY BE

When thoughts become crushing, and sadness or other feelings dominate, pause. Breathe slowly and deeply. Rather than reacting to the unpleasant experience, allow yourself to slow down and observe what you are thinking, how you are feeling, and the physical sensations in your body. Notice without judging or labeling. Tell yourself, "Right now I'm feeling _____." While allowing these thoughts, feelings, and sensations, shift your attention and, with curiosity, explore what else you might be experiencing. Is there a glimmer of pride that you are doing this exercise? A touch of gratitude about something? Tell yourself, "And right now I'm also feeling _____."

GO BACK TO the latest negative thought you pondered on page 35. Now, shift your attention *away* from the negative thought and describe what else was happening when it was last on your mind. Use all of your senses to vividly picture the situation. What did you see? Hear? Smell? Feel (think of the temperature, air movement, and textures)? Can you recall details now that you didn't actively notice originally?

WHAT WOULD IT be like to experience a situation neutrally, paying attention to the details of the moment instead of your thoughts? What effect would this have on your emotions? Would you do anything differently?

PAUSE FOR A MINDFUL BITE

The renowned mindfulness teacher Thích Nhất Hạnh speaks of eating mindfully, rather than on autopilot. Instead of distracted eating, which keeps you lost in thoughts or external distractions, with mindful eating, you fully experience your food—and the act of eating—by directing your attention to what you're doing.

Mindful eating takes practice, so ease into it. Choose a favorite healthy food (ideally, something you can easily eat with your fingers), and mindfully eat just one bite. Start a mindful eating practice with this simple exercise, and gradually expand it over time.

- Pick up your snack. Take in its color and notice all the little nuances and details.
- Bring it to your nose and inhale. What does it smell like? Describe it to yourself.
- Feel its texture, temperature, and weight. Does anything stand out?
- Take one bite, noticing the experience of biting into it. What is the texture like? How does it taste?
- Pay attention and savor it as you slowly chew and feel the sensation as you swallow.

LOOK BACK AT some of your earlier responses, especially the lists of thoughts you jotted down in the first prompt that led you to pick up this journal. Although your journey has just begun, do you notice a shift in your perspective as your awareness of the nature of your thoughts has grown?

MINDFUL MOVEMENT: GENTLE STRETCHING

Practices such as yoga, tai chi, and mindful walking allow you to unite mind and body. Moving and stretching promote health and well-being, and paying attention to it offers another way to pull yourself out of the thoughts and feelings that bog you down in depression. Of course, our bodies are unique to each of us, and there is no "right" or "wrong" way to move. Physical limitations don't reflect our inherent worth and value. Please honor your own body and move, or ask others to help you move, in ways that work for you. (See the Resources on page 172 for information on HelpGuide, which offers ways to move with limited mobility, and always check with your doctor before embarking on an exercise or yoga stretching practice to ensure you move in ways that are healthy for your body.)

- Sit at the edge of a chair with your back straight and your feet flat on the floor.
- Inhale slowly as you twist gently to place both hands on the outside of your left leg.
- Exhale slowly as you twist gently to the other side.
- Repeat several times and notice how you feel.

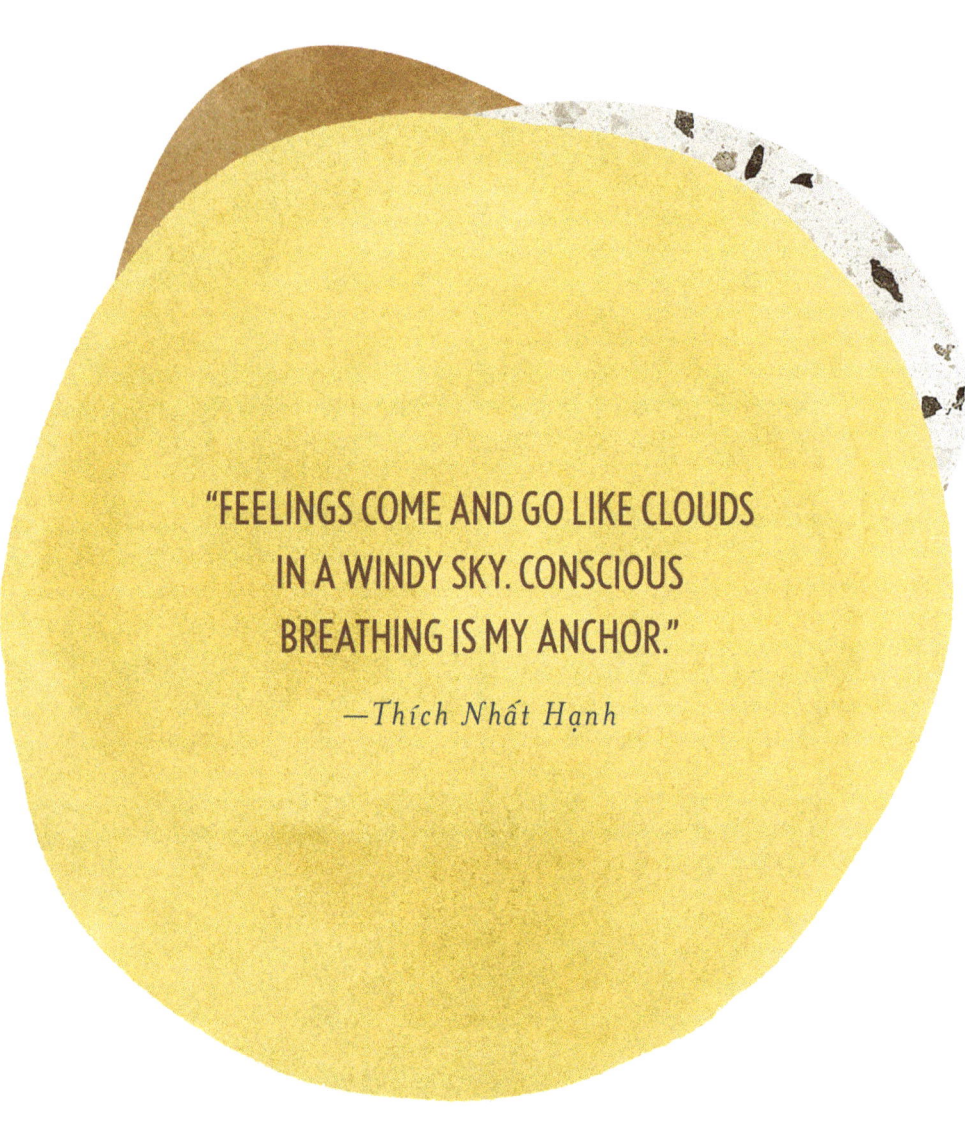

"FEELINGS COME AND GO LIKE CLOUDS IN A WINDY SKY. CONSCIOUS BREATHING IS MY ANCHOR."

—*Thích Nhất Hạnh*

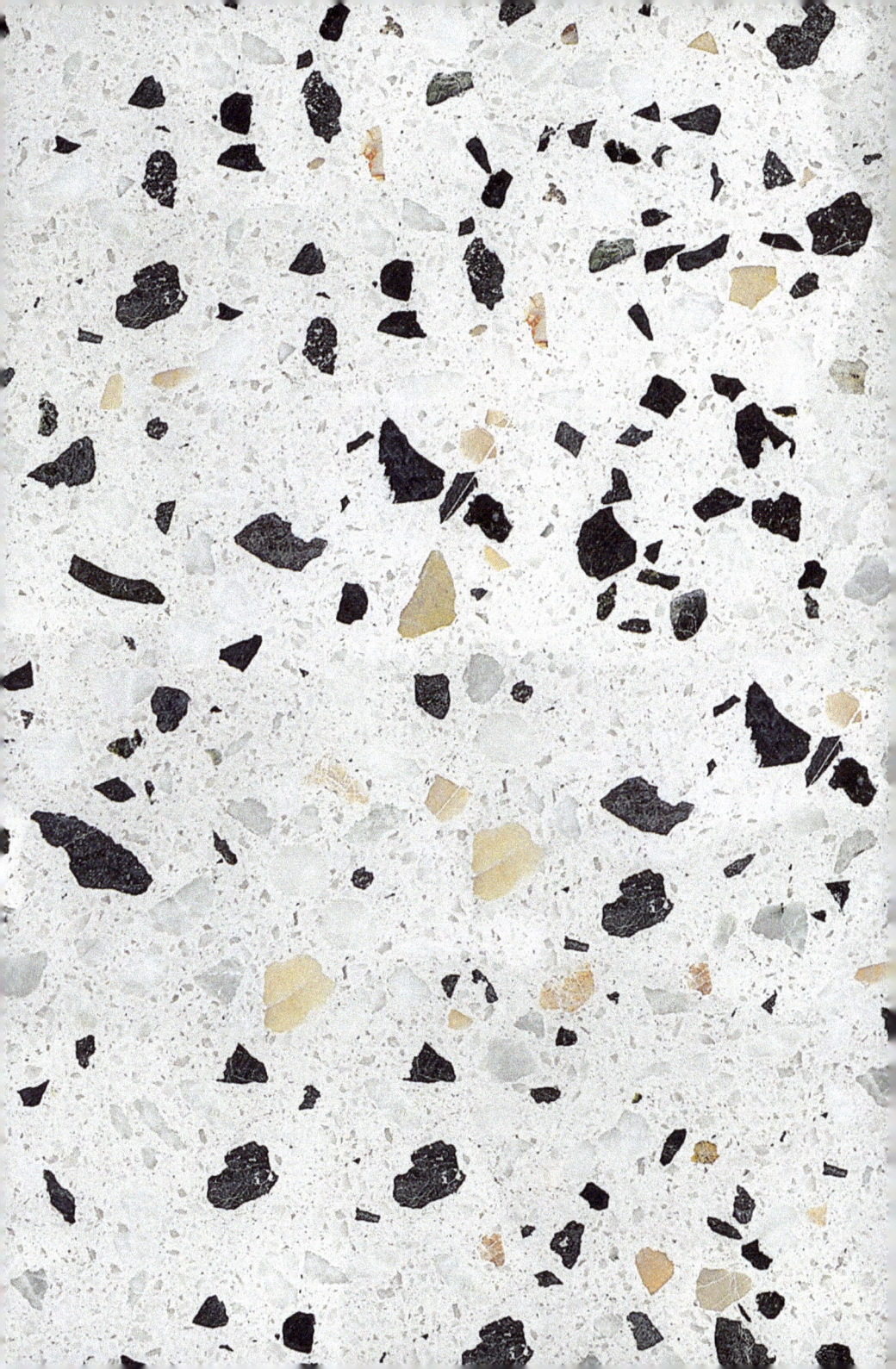

Notice, But Don't Dwell

In completing part 1, you've begun to increase your insight into your thoughts, emotions, and innate reactions to situations. That burgeoning sense of awareness lights the way along the path to forming a new relationship with yourself, your thoughts and feelings, and your life.

Would you be surprised to learn that one effective way to overcome depression is not to try to get rid of it? Bear with me here! Because your brain has a natural tendency to generate negative thoughts, it is okay to have these negative thoughts and feelings. It's an unrealistic goal to *never* feel down, empty, angry, irritable, or anything else that your experience with depression makes you feel. Instead, the ultimate goal is to live a healthier, happier life by forming a different relationship with your negative thoughts.

The more you focus on those thoughts, feelings, and situations and treat them as if they're facts, the deeper depression's hooks can sink into you. But by noticing your automatic thoughts and feelings, you can put some space between yourself and depression.

In this conscious space, you can notice your thoughts with openness and curiosity, observing them without judgment. Being mindful and staying present in each moment, as we'll explore in part 2, is very liberating. Rather than holding on to problems, trying to ignore them, or attempting to make them go away, when you are mindful, you can accept your thoughts and feelings without letting them consume you.

BECOME AN OBSERVER of your own experience. Recall a recent difficult situation. Name or describe your reaction to it: your thoughts, emotions, and body sensations.

Look back at what you just wrote. Circle anything that involves a judgment or a belief imposed on the situation. (For example, consider these statements: "I was too tired to go to my daughter's game. I'm a terrible parent." Here, you would circle "terrible parent," because that is an evaluation of your ability to parent.)

NOW, REVIEW THOSE circled words and phrases. These judgments are often a source of misery, and sticking to them leads to continued suffering. Accepting a situation for what it is helps you let it drift away rather than ruminating over it. Rewrite your circled judgments here to make them more neutral. ("Terrible parent" might become "a parent who made a mistake" or "a parent who cares deeply.")

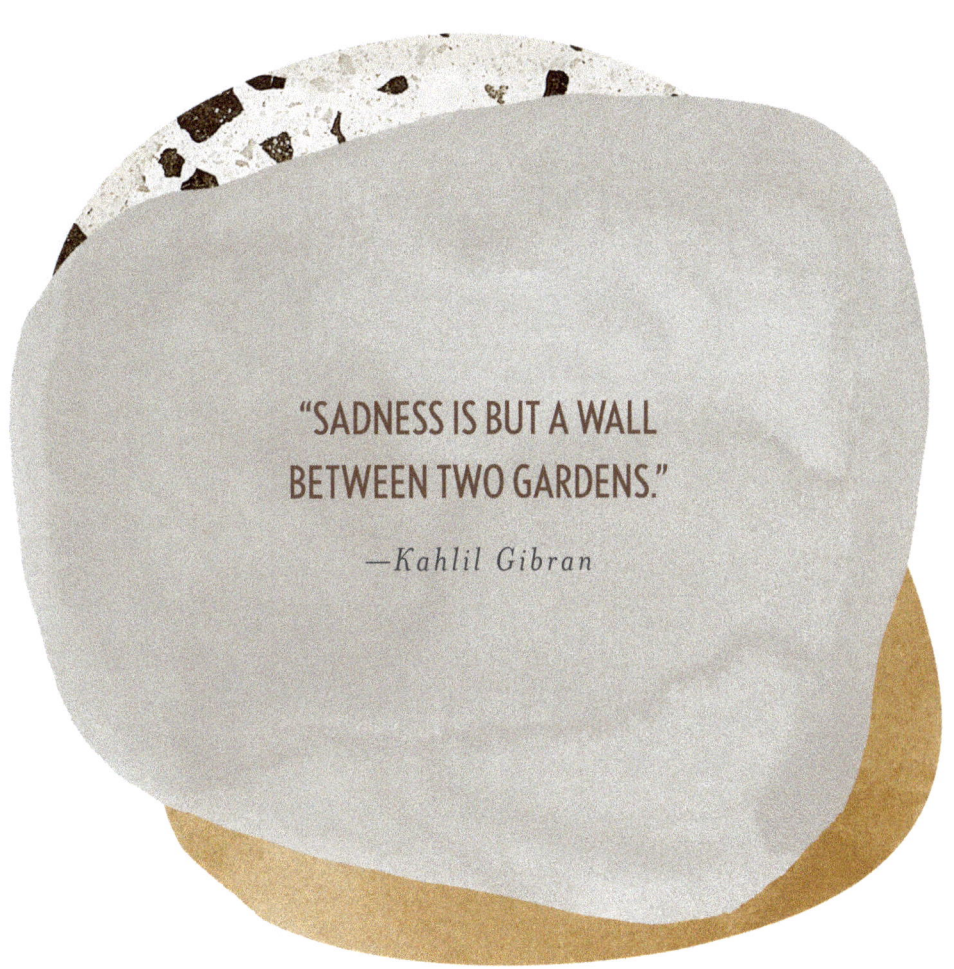

"SADNESS IS BUT A WALL BETWEEN TWO GARDENS."

—*Kahlil Gibran*

DEPRESSION MAKES IT difficult to accept yourself as you are. Depression is a bully that turns people against themselves. Become mindfully aware of yourself (how you *really* are, not how depression sees you) and describe yourself as you are in this moment.

SHIFTING OUT OF AUTOPILOT

Many times you operate on autopilot, simply going through the motions of your day while your thoughts spin off in many different directions, often cascading downward and pulling you along with them. You don't have to actively force a change. Simply begin to become aware of when you are lost in thought and not paying attention to what you are doing in the moment. When you catch yourself, gently return your concentration to one aspect of the present moment (a sight, sound, scent, texture, sensation, or person you're with).

TAKE THREE SLOW, deep breaths, and pay attention to the experience of breathing, the sound, and the feel of air entering and leaving your body. Do you notice any changes in your thoughts, emotions, and body sensations afterward? Maybe you feel a bit lighter or a little less tense. Perhaps you are thinking about different things. If so, jot down what you observe.

ON A SCALE from 1 to 10, with 1 representing "not at all" and 10 representing "completely," to what extent were you able to keep your attention exclusively on your breath (without your mind wandering) when you took those three slow, deep breaths?

not at all ① ② ③ ④ ⑤ ⑥ ⑦ ⑧ ⑨ ⑩ *completely*

Now, note any thoughts or frustrations that came up.

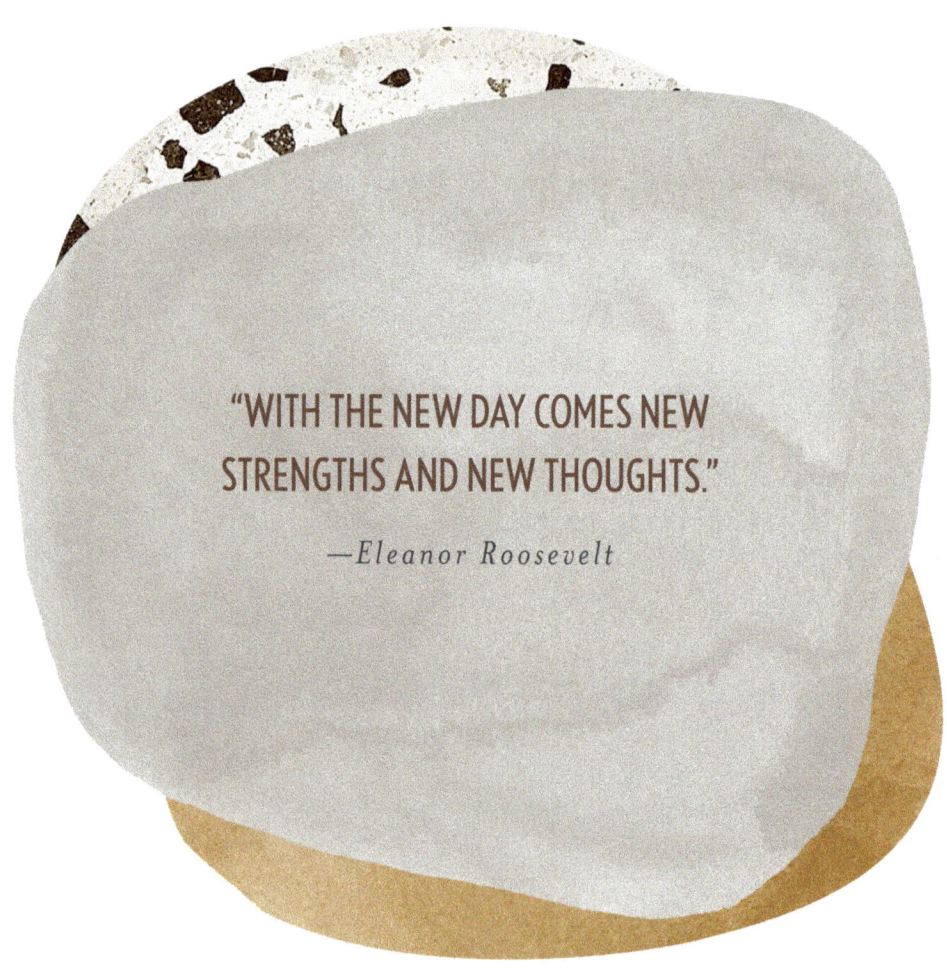

"WITH THE NEW DAY COMES NEW STRENGTHS AND NEW THOUGHTS."

—Eleanor Roosevelt

THE HUMAN BRAIN is a wandering brain. Mindfulness exercises like tuning into your breathing are not about emptying your mind; they're about increasing your awareness of your wandering thoughts and improving your ability to redirect your attention when it wanders. Describe what it will be like when you start catching your wandering thoughts and returning your attention to something in the moment, such as a favorite photo, a vibrant plant, or the scent of a candle.

MINDFULNESS SIGNALS

Being on autopilot robs you of living fully in the moment because you're constantly focused on your thoughts and feelings. It's tricky at first to catch yourself on autopilot, so to gently encourage yourself to shift into *this* moment, pepper your living space with signals to remind you to let go of negative emotions and settle into the moment. On sticky notes, draw pictures of what mindful living means to you (you might draw a blooming flower, a shining sun, or some stick figures to represent you and your loved ones). Place them in random places like your wallet, a desk drawer, the refrigerator, the place you keep your keys, on the steering wheel of your car, near the TV remote, and under the sink with the dish soap. When you encounter a signal, notice your thoughts and shift your awareness to the current moment.

DEPRESSION TELLS YOU stories about everything that is wrong with you and your life. It fills your mind with a world of wrongs and then it holds you trapped there. Close your eyes and imagine your trap, picturing it in detail. Describe what this trap is like for you.

HERE'S A SECRET that depression doesn't want you to know: You feel like a captive, but in reality, you aren't shackled in your mind or locked behind a door. This trap exists, but it is separate from you and other experiences. Turn your attention to what is around you right now that *isn't* your trap, and describe it in detail, calling on all of your senses to fully experience it.

WHEN YOU'RE AWARE that depression's ability to make you feel trapped is just one experience among many, you're able to wander, noticing and experiencing other things. Where would you like to go? Who will be there? What will you be like when you're there?

BREATHE IN COLOR

Depression is colorless. Truly. Depression affects how you perceive the world and can make everything look dull and flat. Use this mindful breathing exercise to positively affect your nervous system and begin to put the color back in your life from the inside out.

- Close your eyes and imagine a bright, vivid rainbow arching over you.
- Slowly inhale the color red. Imagine it filling your body.
- Slowly exhale the color orange, giving the gift of color to the world around you.
- Inhale again, slowly breathing in yellow.
- Exhale green and imagine it saturating your surroundings.
- Breathe in, filling yourself with electric blue light.
- Breathe out, filling your world with radiant purple.

PICK ONE NEGATIVE thought about yourself that frequently plays in your mind. Write it here, off to the side. Let that thought just exist on this page while, in the rest of the space, you describe yourself in ways that have nothing to do with this thought.

REREAD THE DESCRIPTION you just wrote. Put a huge star by three descriptions that make you feel proud. Why do these particular items evoke a sense of self-respect? This helps you increase your awareness of your whole self.

LOOK BACK AND celebrate your progress! Flip back to page 2 and see what you wrote. How are your thoughts a little different now? Scribble some happy drawings to cheer yourself on!

MEET YOUR THOUGHTS AND FEELINGS WITH CURIOSITY

The human brain is constantly thinking, coming up with things that you now know aren't always true. Observe these thoughts as if you were watching a dance. Don't intentionally zoom in on one of the "dancers," but if you do catch yourself following a particular thought or emotion, meet it with curiosity rather than judgment. Rather than hating the thought, trying to change it, or berating yourself, simply notice it with open curiosity: *Where is it going next? What if it were wrong? Oh, this thought says I'm worthless. Okay. I'm going to see what other dancers are like. Hmm.* Can you begin to appreciate your mind for its ability to drum up automatic negative thoughts?

It may seem odd to thank your mind for having negative thoughts. Remember that about 70 percent of thoughts are negative. Your brain watches for problems to keep you out of danger. It is also highly creative and able to think in complex ways. Appreciating your brain's efforts helps you develop a nonjudgmental perspective and helps you stop being so hard on yourself for having thoughts.

DEPRESSION CAN MAKE it feel impossible to do things or go places, in part because your thoughts and feelings about a situation, such as work or being around other people in a social setting, have a habit of arriving early—before you even physically arrive in that place. Describe a time when you anticipated bad things about a situation before it happened.

REGARDING THE SITUATION you just described, what thoughts did you have? How did you feel before you arrived? How did you feel when you were there? Did these pre-judgments affect or color your actions somehow?

THINK OF SOMEWHERE you have to go or something you have to do. Instead of your mind arriving before you and creating negative judgments, imagine that you are brand new to it, a beginner. You've never before experienced it, so you have no judgments to make. Describe this place or event from this open mindset.

MOVE IN A MINDFUL WAY

Do this indoors or outside. Depression is heavy and exhausting and can make any exercise daunting. If you're battling fatigue or soreness, make your first mindful walks brief, just a minute or a few steps out the door and back. The key is to move your body and pay attention to your experience.

Begin by placing both feet firmly on the ground. Wiggle your toes and feel your feet in your shoes or directly on the ground or floor. Step your left foot forward and then your right. As you step, focus your attention by staying to yourself, "Left. Right." If you are still walking after a few steps, turn your attention to your surroundings. Note sights by naming them. If you catch yourself judging ("That's an ugly car," or, "I can't concentrate on just one thing. I'm terrible at this."), just say to yourself, "Judging." Return to noticing sights. Gradually expand your attention to focus on sounds, smells, and then sensations, like the feel of the air on your skin, the temperature of the room, or the feel of an object between your fingers.

If you get around differently, perhaps in a wheelchair, or have difficulty walking, you can tailor this mindfulness exercise to suit you. You can move in your own way, or you can even sit in one place and focus on one particular sense. Look around appreciatively and focus on pleasing sights, sounds, or smells.

FROM THIS POSITION of openness (often called "beginner's mind") you explored on page 67, become curious about your thoughts. Are you jumping to conclusions? Are you assuming thoughts are facts? Are you imposing impossible standards on yourself or the situation?

CURIOSITY ALLOWS YOU to expand your thinking beyond problems to possibilities. Notice what is on your mind right now. Ask yourself, "What else?" Without trying to force changes, let whatever is on your mind just now be there, and list it here.

DEPRESSION IS UNCOMFORTABLE, so it's very natural to want to resist or avoid it. About how much time do you spend thinking about your experience with depression?

a. I think about it a lot. It's on my mind pretty much all the time, no matter what I'm doing.
b. Honestly, I'm often not sure what I'm thinking about because my brain is foggy or full of a lot of different things or empty.
c. I never think about it.

Becoming aware of the tendencies toward struggle and avoidance helps release you from the hooks of depression. Awareness leads to acceptance. Don't worry—I'm not asking you to give in to depression. Acceptance means that rather than tangling with thoughts and emotions, you let go of them so you have room for other things. If you no longer held on to bothersome beliefs, what would you have room for?

LIST FOUR OR five things you don't want to accept. These can be thoughts, feelings, or situations/events. Be specific. If your first thought is "depression," encourage yourself to go a little bit deeper. What is it about depression (or whatever else you've chosen here) that you don't want to accept?

STUDY YOUR LIST. How, exactly, are these things affecting your relationships with yourself, your loved ones, others, and your life itself? Are they preventing you from enjoying certain situations? Are you missing out on your time with loved ones because you're not fully present with them? Are these things clouding the way you interpret what others are saying? These are just some examples. Get personal, and notice what is going on for you and your life.

MINDFUL MOVEMENT: FORWARD FOLD

In yoga, the forward fold is used to release tension throughout the body and promote flexibility. Numerous studies have found that practicing yoga helps reduce stress, depression, and anxiety because it impacts the spine and nervous system. Pause and do a forward fold often throughout your day.

- Stand tall, with your feet about hip-width apart, arms at your sides.
- Slowly, and with your knees slightly bent, fold forward, letting your hands dangle toward the floor. You don't have to touch the floor. Only go as far as is comfortable.
- Hold the stretch for three breaths.
- Slowly roll up to standing.

If a forward fold isn't something that is part of the way you move, that's okay. The key is to somehow tune in to your body to shift your thoughts and energy away from the challenges or frustrations that may be running through your mind. You might squeeze your hands into fists and release the tension, but if that causes pain or you are otherwise unable to do this, perhaps you want to notice your breathing and count your inhalations and exhalations. Remember, too, to check the Resources section (page 172) for information on exercising while keeping limitations in mind.

KNOWING THAT WHAT you focus on is what grows, what might happen if you noticed unpleasant thoughts, feelings, and situations and accepted their presence so you could turn your attention to something else?

ONE WAY TO shift your attention and slip off depression's hook is to savor what you are doing in the moment, no matter what that is. Practice this now. Write down one negative thought or problem. Become curious. What else is going on in your moment (what's around you, who are you with, etc.)? Write down one thing. Experience this other thing fully and savor it. Describe the little details of what you see and feel. Do you hear, smell, or taste anything?

BODY SCAN ON THE GO

Depression appears in both body and mind. Tune in to your body regularly to catch signals that your mind is hooked on negative thoughts and emotions. Wherever you are, periodically scan your body and breathe to reset. Notice your feet, your lower legs, your knees, your upper legs, your gut and everything inside, your chest, your shoulders, arms, elbows, wrists and hands, your neck, your face, your head. Locate areas of tension and, while concentrating on these areas, inhale deeply and exhale slowly. Tune in to the subtle shift in mind and body. Is there a subtle change in your mood or physical sensations?

NEGATIVE THOUGHTS AND emotions can sometimes dominate the human mind, but there's lots of room for positive ideas and feelings, too. But depression makes them hard to spot. Let your gaze fall on something pleasing, like a nearby object, photo, person, or pet. Describe what you've chosen, with sensory details.

JOT DOWN THE positive thoughts, emotions, and sensations that surfaced when you were describing this pleasing object, person, or pet. When you're aware of the negative, you can practice allowing it to exist and shifting your attention to the positive.

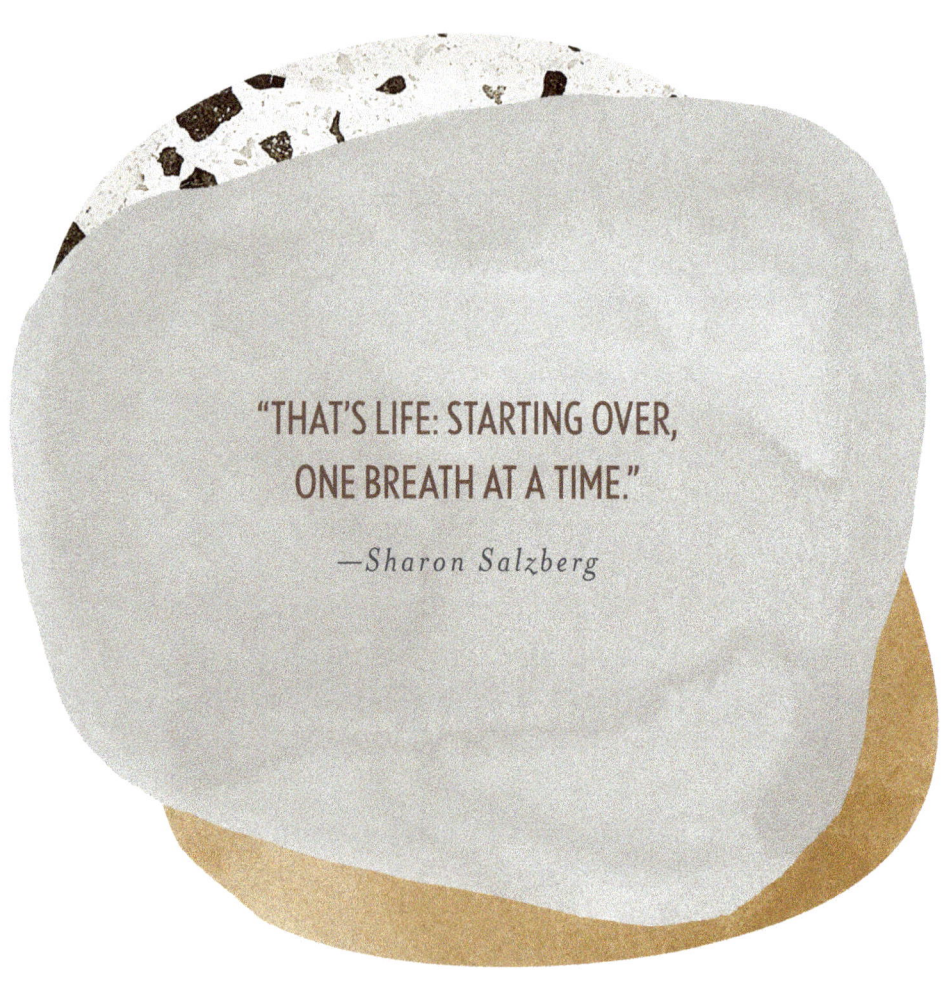

"THAT'S LIFE: STARTING OVER, ONE BREATH AT A TIME."

—*Sharon Salzberg*

DEPRESSION CAN BE exhausting. You may feel like you don't have energy to work through it and simply want to resign yourself to it. You're using this journal, so that means that even if you're utterly fatigued, you're finding the strength to move forward anyway. Write a letter of appreciation to yourself for this. End your letter by reminding yourself why you're persevering and going on this journey.

IN THE VERY first prompt of part 2 (page 46), you began to observe your experiences by thinking about a difficult situation and describing your reaction. Look back on that now. If you were to experience that situation again, how would your reaction be different? Describe your new thoughts, feelings, and sensations. Acknowledge how far you've come!

OPENNESS TO WHAT IS

Openness and acceptance are skills that can be learned, developed, and honed. Use this exercise to prime your whole self—mind and body—for acceptance.

- Sit or lie down comfortably.
- Place a hand on your belly and one on your heart.
- Tell yourself, "I'm open to all my different experiences today."
- Wiggle your arms and hands.
- Say, "I embrace the positive things in what I'm experiencing right now, in this moment."
- Touch your head and roll it around.
- Say, "My mind is open to new things."

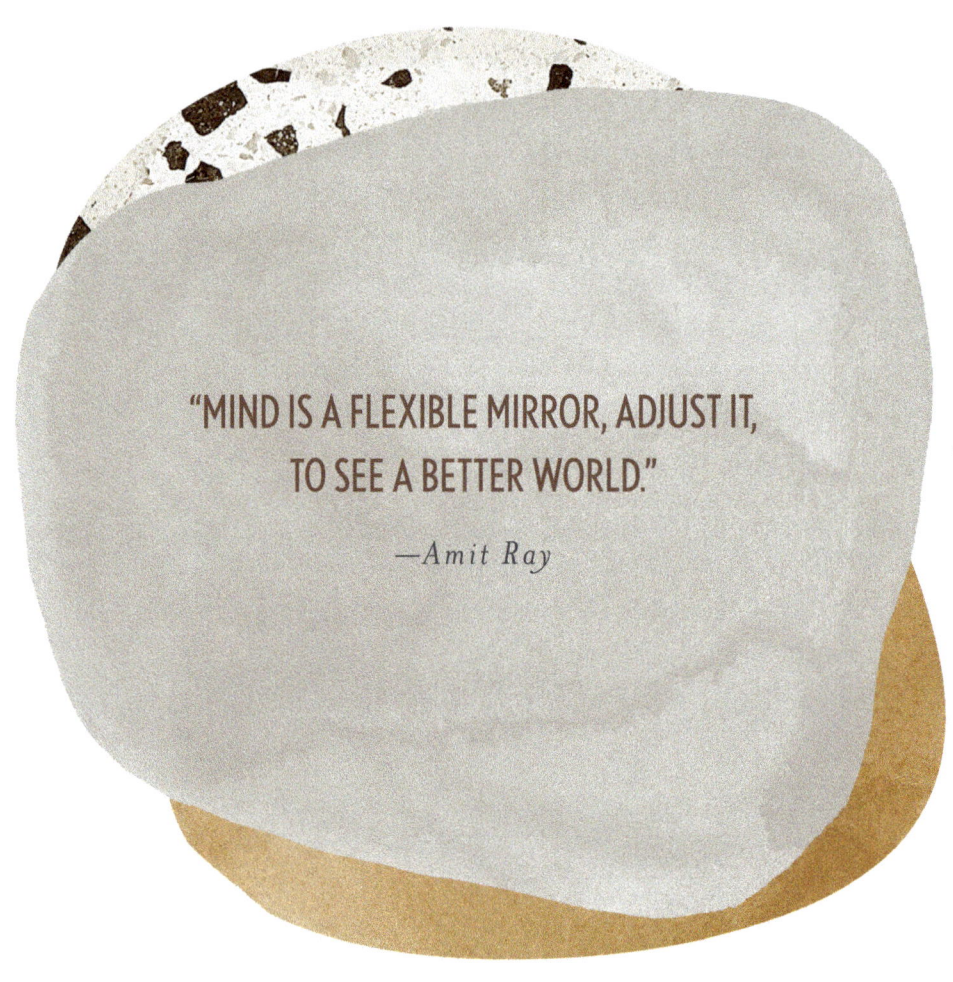

"MIND IS A FLEXIBLE MIRROR, ADJUST IT, TO SEE A BETTER WORLD."

—*Amit Ray*

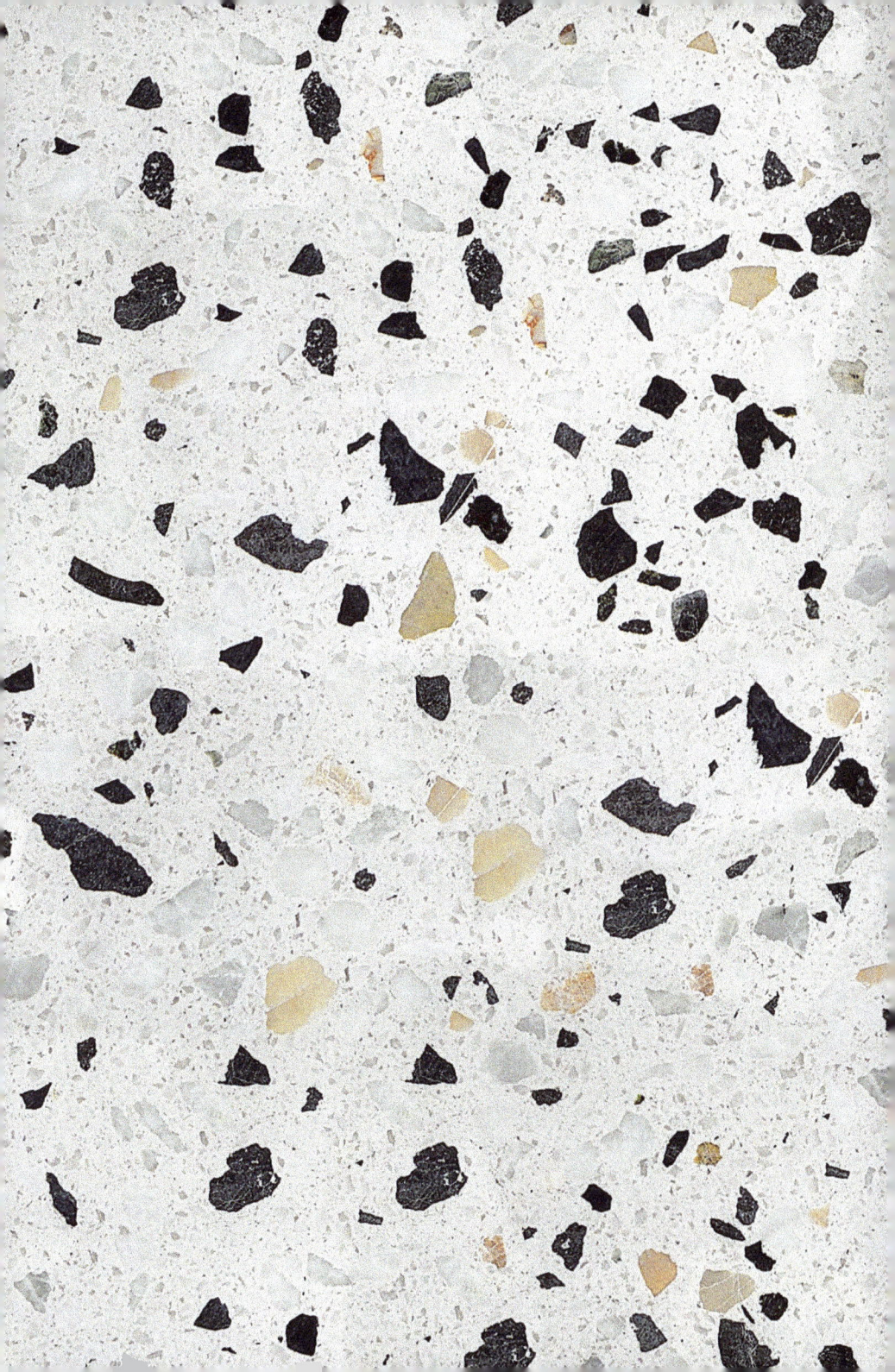

Depression Doesn't Define Me

Here's a truth that depression doesn't want you to know: Depression isn't *you*. It isn't who you are at your core. It has absolutely nothing to do with your strengths, gifts, unique qualities, personality, or values. Depression is merely something you happen to be experiencing right now in your life.

I know that to say that depression is "merely" an experience probably doesn't feel right, at least not at first. The experience of depression quite likely looms large and feels oppressive in your life. I compare it to a boulder that is not only blocking your path forward but has rolled on top of you, blocking your view of the possibilities that exist beyond it—including what is truly within you. Depression can be all-encompassing and usurps your thoughts, emotions, body, and actions, which is why it makes sense that you lose sight of yourself when experiencing it.

In part 3, you will begin to peer past depression and your symptoms to see who you really are at your core. For many people, depression obscures the memory of who they are and twists it, inserting negative beliefs and guilty feelings. As you work through this part and integrate the practices into your life, you will empower yourself to re-emerge. You'll start to separate yourself from the experience of depression so you can gradually come out from under its weight.

DEPRESSION CAN CAUSE deep self-doubt, guilt, and feelings of worthlessness. Although it can be unpleasant, acknowledging these emotions allows you to face and move past them. What does depression try to tell you about yourself? Describe your thoughts and feelings about yourself using words or by drawing a picture.

IN WHAT WAYS does your negative self-talk—your thoughts and feelings about yourself—limit your life?

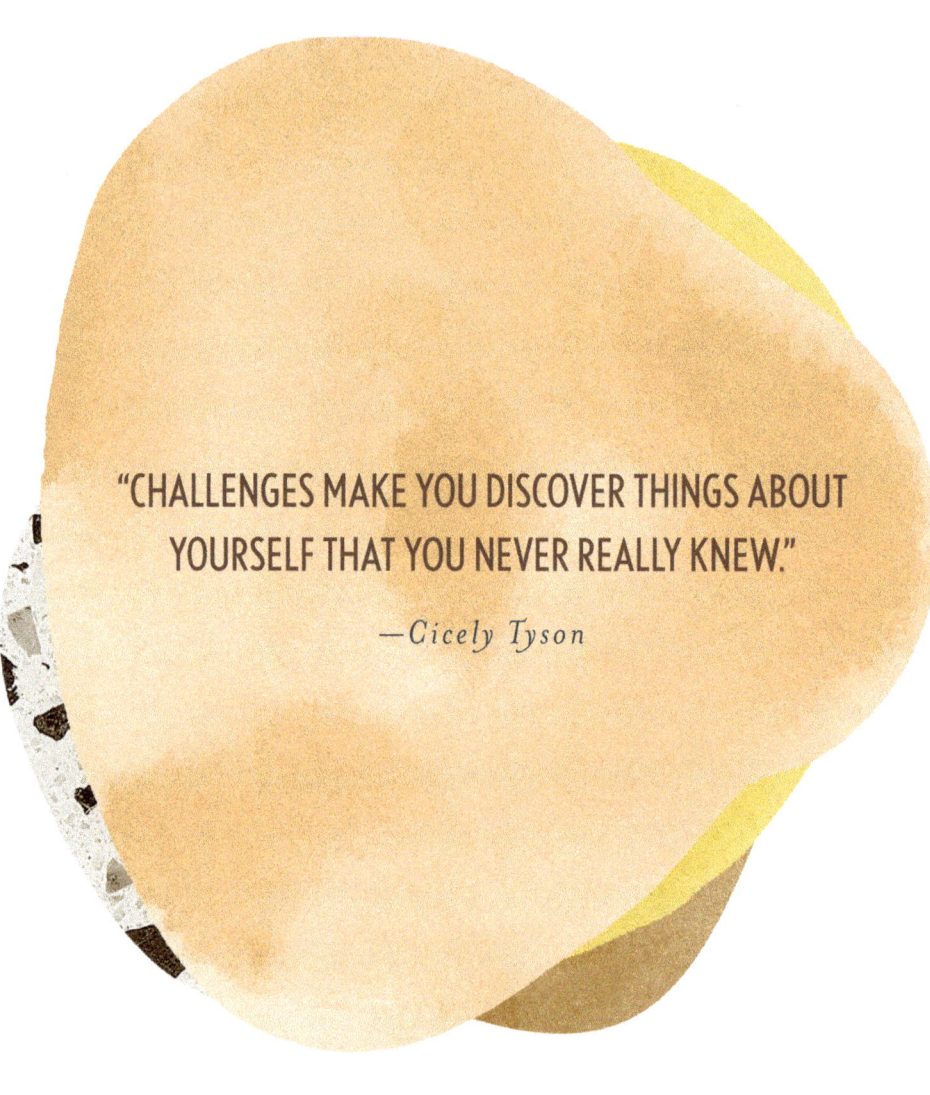

"CHALLENGES MAKE YOU DISCOVER THINGS ABOUT YOURSELF THAT YOU NEVER REALLY KNEW."

—*Cicely Tyson*

TO EMERGE FROM underneath the boulder of depression, practice catching yourself being mean to yourself and switching gears. Reread your list of descriptions about what depression tells you about yourself (page 88), and select four of them. Rewrite them in a neutral way rather than in harsh, absolute self-judgments. (For example, "I ruin everything," might become, "Like everyone, I make mistakes sometimes.")

ONE FOOT IN FRONT OF THE OTHER

You might feel as though you're too depleted to do what it takes to overcome depression. That normal feeling is part of depression—it doesn't represent your ability to take charge of your life. You don't have to wait until you have energy in order to begin; in fact, taking small actions every day, like writing in this journal, will gradually increase your energy so you can do more and more. Knowing your *why*, your reason for beating depression, can encourage you to keep going, despite feeling exhausted.

Complete this sentence: "I am working to beat depression because _____."

Write your answer on a sheet of paper or text it to yourself, and reread it every morning when you wake up, in the afternoon, and in the evening before bed.

INSTEAD OF BEING caught up in the thoughts you explored on page 88, what would it be like to acknowledge them and then shift your attention? List as many things as you can to complete this sentence: "If I shifted my thoughts instead of remaining stuck in them, thinking about them over and over again, I would feel _____ and I could be/do/have _____."

THERE ARE SO many things to pay attention to instead of the negative self-talk that depression plays on loop. Make a list of the sights, sounds, smells, textures, tastes, and events that you could shift your attention to again and again when depression's negative voice ramps up.

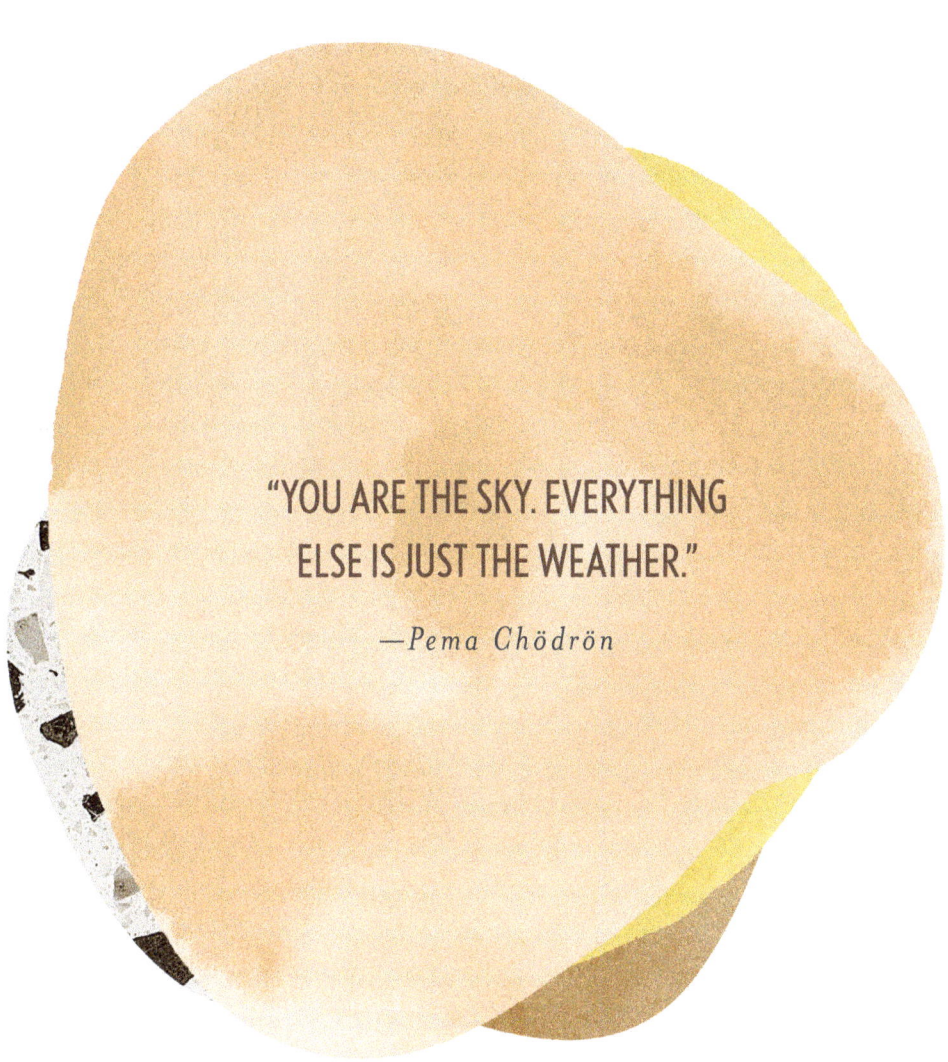

"YOU ARE THE SKY. EVERYTHING ELSE IS JUST THE WEATHER."

—*Pema Chödrön*

THE SKY IS steady. It is what it is even when stormy weather rolls in. (Above the clouds, the sky remains constantly blue.) You are like this. Depression is only a storm that has blown in. Look past those things that depression makes you think about yourself, and describe the qualities that make you *you*.

TIME TO PAUSE and appreciate how far you've come! At the beginning of part 2, you wrote about a difficult situation and your associated thoughts, feelings, and body sensations (page 46). Look back on that now. Although the situation itself hasn't changed, what new thoughts and emotions do you have about it? Does it cause the same reaction in your body as it first did?

ASK YOURSELF "AND WHAT ELSE?"

Open your mind to your full, vibrant self—the real you behind the experience of depression. When you find yourself caught up in negative self-talk, expand your awareness by asking, "And what else?" Doing so allows you to untangle yourself from depression's intricate web because you're neither buying in to depression's narrow view of yourself nor making it stronger by focusing on it. For example, if you find yourself thinking something harsh like, "I'm lazy and worthless," immediately ask, "And what else?" Then, answer the question with descriptions of what you're good at or a reminder of something you accomplished today (it can be anything, even standing up and stretching).

WRITE A LETTER of gratitude to yourself, showing yourself appreciation for all that you are and what you do. "Dear Me, _____."

NOW, HOW ABOUT writing a letter of gratitude to depression? You don't have to love depression! But shifting your thoughts about it helps you slip away from its strong grasp. Maybe it has given you a deeper appreciation for the times when you feel better, or perhaps it is motivating you to grow. "Dear Depression, _____."

REREAD YOUR LETTERS of gratitude to yourself and to depression and look for patterns. What do you notice about yourself? Are you someone who can see a bigger picture? Do you have abilities you haven't fully appreciated? Do you have new goals because of depression?

BE MINDFUL OF THE REAL YOU

Use this mindful body scan to increase your awareness of your true self.

- Sit or lie down comfortably, with your spine straight and muscles relaxed.
- Take a few slow, deep breaths, feeling your stomach expand as you inhale and contract as you exhale. Reflect on the following aspects of gratitude and body joy you have for yourself.
- Turn your attention to your lower body. *Feet and legs, I'm grateful that we courageously go places even if we have limits.*
- Move your focus to your gut. *Belly, even if my appetite is off, thank you for digesting what I eat to nourish me.*
- Concentrate on your arms. *Thank you for helping me show my love with warm embraces.*
- Check in with your neck. *Neck, my head is heavy and can be hard to hold. Thank you for your strength.*
- Proceed to your head. *Brain, thank you for functioning and persevering through depression. I'm grateful that you're helping me find my true self. Thank you for my ability to turn my attention to new things every moment.*

DEPRESSION TAKES THE excitement out of life, zapping your passion and turning everything dull or too exhausting to bother with. Beyond this storm cloud, though, your zest for life still radiates. Make a list of activities you would do, places you would go, and people you'd connect with if depression wasn't holding you back.

MORE THAN ONE CHAPTER

Depression has a way of making it seem like it is your life. In truth, depression is one experience in your life—not your full story. Think of every moment as a blank page full of opportunities. Make it a habit to pause and ask yourself how your book is going and whether it's time to turn the page and start a brand-new chapter. Consider setting an alarm to sound hourly to break yourself out of autopilot, habitually rereading the same chapter of yourself dictated by your depression. When it chimes, look away from your current page and ask yourself, "What do I see, hear, smell, feel, and taste? How do I want *this* page of my story to read?"

CONSIDER THE QUALITIES you have deep inside that will allow you to do what you used to love. Write them here. Maybe you love learning new things or enjoy the feeling that comes from doing small acts of kindness—even if you can't do them right now, they're still part of you.

WRITE ABOUT A time when you were at your best. What was happening? How did you act? How did you feel?

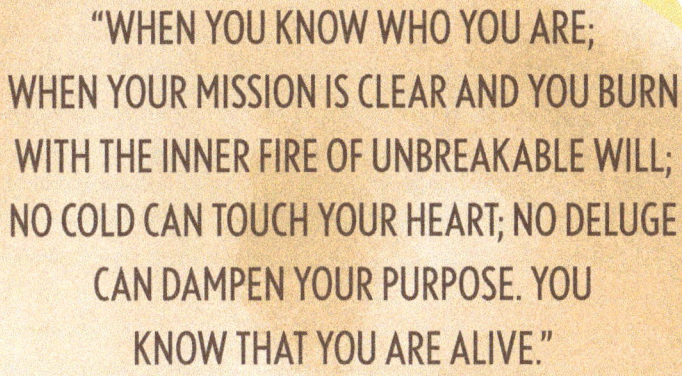

"WHEN YOU KNOW WHO YOU ARE; WHEN YOUR MISSION IS CLEAR AND YOU BURN WITH THE INNER FIRE OF UNBREAKABLE WILL; NO COLD CAN TOUCH YOUR HEART; NO DELUGE CAN DAMPEN YOUR PURPOSE. YOU KNOW THAT YOU ARE ALIVE."

—*Chief Seattle (Si'ahl)
of the Suquamish and
Duwamish Tribes*

DESPITE WHAT DEPRESSION might say, you have many character strengths. The VIA Institute on Character has identified 24 primary strengths that all humans possess. Although everyone possesses all of them, we have them in different degrees (that's what makes us all unique). Consider this list of character strengths, and circle your own top five. A hint: Which ones make you feel a bit more energized or excited, even if you don't actually have the energy right now to take action?

- Appreciation of beauty and excellence
- Bravery
- Creativity
- Curiosity
- Fairness
- Forgiveness
- Gratitude
- Honesty
- Hope
- Humility
- Humor
- Judgment
- Kindness
- Leadership
- Love
- Love of learning
- Perseverance
- Perspective
- Prudence
- Self-regulation
- Social intelligence
- Spirituality
- Teamwork
- Zest

DAILY STRENGTHS PRACTICE

Your strengths are part of you, and you can use them to create the life you want and to shape your thoughts, feelings, and actions. Recall your top strengths. Choose one of them, and brainstorm ways you can use it mindfully every day. Each week, add another strength to use intentionally in your daily life. (For example, if you choose "Appreciation of Beauty," your list might include such things as stepping outside and observing your favorite tree or flower, noticing the beauty in a loved one and commenting on it, or enjoying a song or work of art.) Think of all the little ways you can use your strength and remember that you can use all of your senses for a richer experience.

ON A SCALE from 1 to 10, with 1 representing "impossible" and 10 representing "effortless," how hard is it for you to identify your strengths? Know that depression makes it extremely difficult for people to see their own strengths. That is why it is so important to spend time identifying and embracing them. Sit with yourself and be honest in this moment.

impossible **1** **2** **3** **4** **5** **6** **7** **8** **9** **10** *effortless*

Using this space, reflect on what makes you strong, considering what others (friends, family, pets, and other loved ones) would say about you.

LIST YOUR TOP five strengths here. Use them to describe yourself in a realistic, positive way. Maybe draw a picture of yourself based on this new description.

HOW DOES THIS description compare to the way you think about yourself when depression has control? What would it be like to think of yourself in terms of your strengths instead of your weaknesses? How would you act? What would your relationships be like? How would you handle problems differently?

STOP AND SMELL THE ROSES

This wise old adage can be powerful. It can pull you out of the automatic negative thoughts and feelings running amok in your mind and into something tangible and concrete in the present moment.

- Choose a real flower, perhaps one that is blooming outside, or close your eyes and imagine a favorite bloom.
- Study it for a moment, concentrating on its color, size, shape, and minute details.
- Bring it to your nose and inhale its scent (real or imagined) slowly and deeply.
- Imagine the fragrance traveling through your whole body, filling you up.
- Exhale completely, imagining the stagnant air of depression leaving your body.
- If scent is not a prominent sense for you, pause and enjoy a flower in another way that is pleasing to you (visually, by touch, and so on).

THINK ABOUT YOURSELF when depression looms over you. Even when it is heaviest, you are living each day no matter how hard it is. Be proud of that! Write about how you are doing it. What is driving you? Focus on what you *are* doing rather than on what you are not.

FORGIVENESS IS A character strength. It doesn't change the past. It does something more powerful; it allows you to let go and move forward. Depression makes self-forgiveness difficult, but you can do it when you approach it with mindful intention. Write a note to yourself offering forgiveness for the mistakes depression holds over you.

DESCRIBE A TIME when you were brave enough to do something difficult, something you didn't think you could do. Did you feel differently after you did it? How?

SAVOR YOUR MEMORIES MINDFULLY

Depression can involve feelings of guilt. In part, this is because it invades your memories and distorts them, twisting them into inaccurate representations of the past. Although it's not helpful to remain stuck in thoughts of the past, reclaiming your memories can be liberating. Begin to notice when you are caught up in negative memories. Acknowledge them, then expand your thoughts and feelings. Recall a fond memory, and bring it to full awareness on your terms. Imagine it neutrally, simply visualizing details about what you saw, the sounds you heard, and nuances of texture and smell. Mentally savor it by observing it without judgment.

DO A MINDFUL self-check-in. What thoughts are on your mind? How do you feel in this moment? What sensations are happening in your body right now? On a scale from 1 to 10, with 1 being the worst and 10 being the best, how would you rate your experience in this moment?

worst ① ② ③ ④ ⑤ ⑥ ⑦ ⑧ ⑨ ⑩ *best*

WHY ISN'T YOUR number one step lower?

WHAT IS ONE thing you could do in this moment that would make your number one step higher?

WHAT STRENGTHS ARE you using to complete this journal?

WHAT OBSTACLES ARE getting in your way as you journey forward? How are you dealing with them? Are you using mindfulness to shift your attention? Are you drawing on your strengths instead of listening to depression's messages? Are you doing something else that helps?

IDENTIFY SOMEONE OR something you love. Describe the person, pet, plant, place, or object here using many of your senses, noting details of appearance, texture, sound, and scent. What would it be like to be mindful with your beloved rather than being lost in thought when you're with them?

WHAT IS MEANINGFUL to you? How can you add more of whatever it is to moments in your life?

YOU'RE OPENING UP and seeing yourself in your own authentic way rather than believing what depression tells you about who you are! Look back to when you first began identifying your strengths and how difficult you rated the activity (page 110). After working through this much of your journal, now how would you rate the difficulty of identifying your strengths? Use the same 1 to 10 scale.

impossible **1** **2** **3** **4** **5** **6** **7** **8** **9** **10** *effortless*

Don't worry—you don't have to be at a 10! Even moving up a single number is progress. What is it like to be mindful and aware of your strengths rather than automatically believing depression's negative self-talk that discounts them?

HAVE TEA WITH YOURSELF (AND TREAT YOURSELF AS AN HONORED GUEST)

The respected Buddhist monk Thích Nhất Hahn speaks of inviting troubles in for tea, remaining fully present in the experience, and just allowing difficult thoughts and emotions to be there rather than engaging in conversation with them. An extension of this is to invite *yourself* for tea, and to treat yourself as an honored, beloved guest. At least once every day, pause to have a cup of tea (or another favorite healthy beverage) with yourself. Use a special mug and sit in a favorite spot. Pay attention to yourself as you would a guest. Experience the moment completely, fully tasting the tea and feeling its warmth fill you. Observe and enjoy your pleasant surroundings. When your thoughts wander, gently return them to your experience with yourself and your tea.

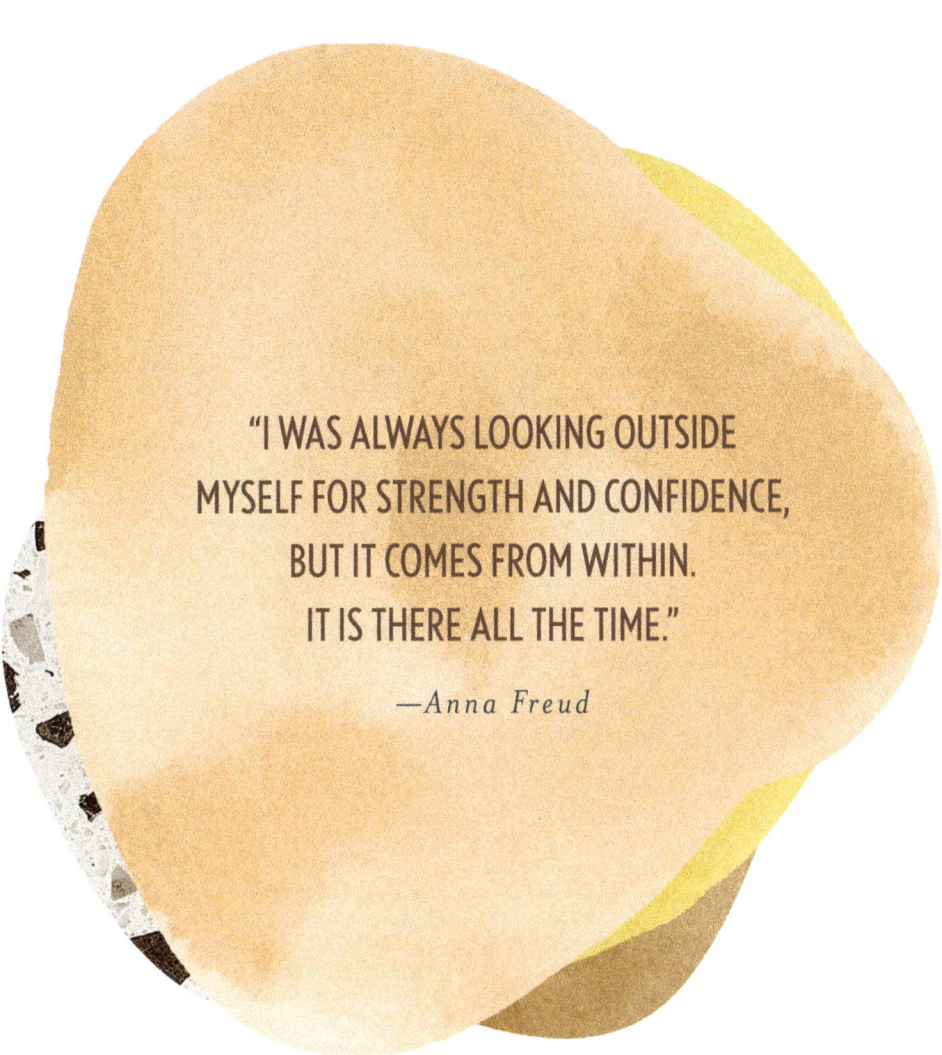

"I WAS ALWAYS LOOKING OUTSIDE MYSELF FOR STRENGTH AND CONFIDENCE, BUT IT COMES FROM WITHIN. IT IS THERE ALL THE TIME."

—*Anna Freud*

The Mindful Way

Mindfulness is so much more than a tool to help you overcome a challenge. It is a way of being with yourself and your world. And with practice, persistence, and patience, it becomes your default way of life, letting depression's disruptions fade. You are able to live a life of balance and ease when negative thoughts are replaced with positivity, gratitude, acceptance, and self-compassion.

Of course, mindfulness doesn't eliminate problems, nor does it make negative thoughts and emotions completely disappear. But as you embrace a more mindful life, you will likely begin to experience a shift away from the mire of depression and toward the tranquility of contentment. You have already begun to know deep truths: Depressive thoughts aren't facts, and you are not defined by depression. You also know how to notice experiences without dwelling within them. Depression is one of your experiences, but there is so much more to you and your textured, varied life than depressive symptoms.

With your concentration on tangible experiences in your present moment instead of focused inward on uncomfortable thoughts and feelings, you are free. You are free to live fully, secure in the knowledge that you no longer need to remain stuck in negative judgments. You are free to choose your response to any difficulty that comes your way. You are free to be your authentic self with your unique strengths and values. The mindful way is the liberated, more lighthearted way. It's how you deserve to live your life.

WHAT MAKES YOU feel energized and alive? You might not experience the energy right now, and that's okay. Think about what has made you feel vibrant in the past.

PREPARE YOURSELF TO do more of what you love by visualizing yourself doing it. Close your eyes and imagine yourself engaging deeply in the activity and successfully completing it. Now, describe the details of what and whom you see, the sounds you hear, the temperature of the room, the scents you notice, the way your muscles feel, the expression on your face, and how you feel/what you think when you have finished it.

AS YOU WROTE about all of the many details of the pleasurable experience, which sense was the easiest for you to call forth? (What did you notice and name most naturally—sights, sounds, smells, or textures/sensations?) How might you use this sense to anchor your attention in any moment when depression symptoms flare?

CONNECT WITH NATURE AND GROW

Numerous studies show that nature is beneficial to our mental health, and it doesn't require fancy gardens or intense trekking through the wilderness. Experience nature and nurture yourself by growing a plant in your living space. The act of taking care of plants has been shown to bring mental health benefits, plus the green addition can be uplifting. For an even bigger boost, appreciate nature mindfully every day, pausing to notice the natural changes and nuances of shape and color, the texture of the leaves, and the earthy scent of the soil.

HOW OFTEN DO you think you could engage in a five-minute visualization like the one on page 131?

a. Once an hour!

b. Once a day, maybe when I first wake up.

c. Three times per week, perhaps on Tuesdays, Thursdays, and Saturdays.

d. Once per week, like on Monday morning to motivate me for the week.

What will be most helpful for you to visualize? Name an experience that you want to have and help yourself picture it by writing your own visualization exercise here. You can use the one you did earlier as a model, or you can create something that feels just right for you. Feel free to focus on just one or two senses or draw on all of them.

HEALTHY HABITS ARE formed with a workable action plan. Which option did you select to indicate how often you could practice a visualization exercise? Write a statement of intention and get specific about exactly when you will practice. (You might write, "I promise myself that I will do my visualization activity every _____ when I _____." Fill in the day(s) of the week and time of day, such as when you wake up or prepare for bed.

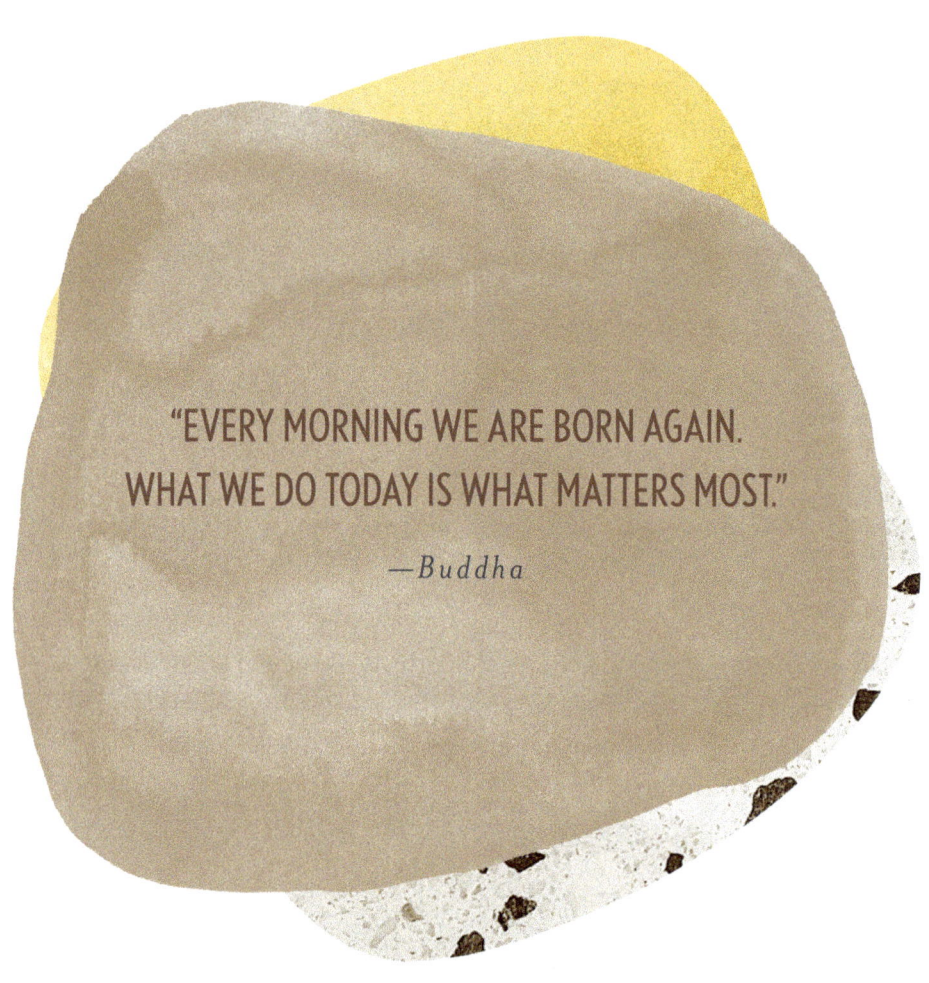

"EVERY MORNING WE ARE BORN AGAIN. WHAT WE DO TODAY IS WHAT MATTERS MOST."

—*Buddha*

WHAT IS ONE small action you can take today to do more of what makes you feel energized and alive? Respond to the following statement: "Today I will _____."

MAKE A LIST of simple, small pleasures you experience in your daily life. (For example, do you love the smell of coffee brewing in the morning, the touch of an animal's fur, or the sight of a favorite picture?)

ACTIVELY EN-JOY MOMENTS

Own your own life by creating little moments of joy every day. Like motivation, joy comes as a result of action. Instead of waiting to feel motivated or happy before you allow yourself to engage in simple pleasures, identify what you like (or used to like), and take simple actions every day to retrain your brain to feel joy and pleasure. If you used to love the outdoors, try opening a window today and enjoying the breeze. Tomorrow, open a door and enjoy the warmth of the sun. The next day, go outside and bask for a few minutes. Small moments of joy lead to even more.

WHAT DOES "JOY" mean to you?

DESCRIBE THREE WAYS you can infuse random moments with joy.

WHAT ABOUT YOUR life makes you feel grateful?

INTENTIONALLY LOOK FOR THE GOOD

Depression clouds what you see and causes you to focus on the negative. What you focus on is what grows, so you can get stuck in a downward spiral of negativity. You can intentionally take back control of what you notice and how you interpret life one moment at a time. Living mindfully helps because it allows you to be present in a moment rather than lost in memories that no longer serve you, such as feelings of guilt about the past. Make it a habit to pause regularly, perhaps setting a timer to chime every 30 or 60 minutes, and look for something good on the spot. Acknowledge it with gratitude and continue with what you were doing.

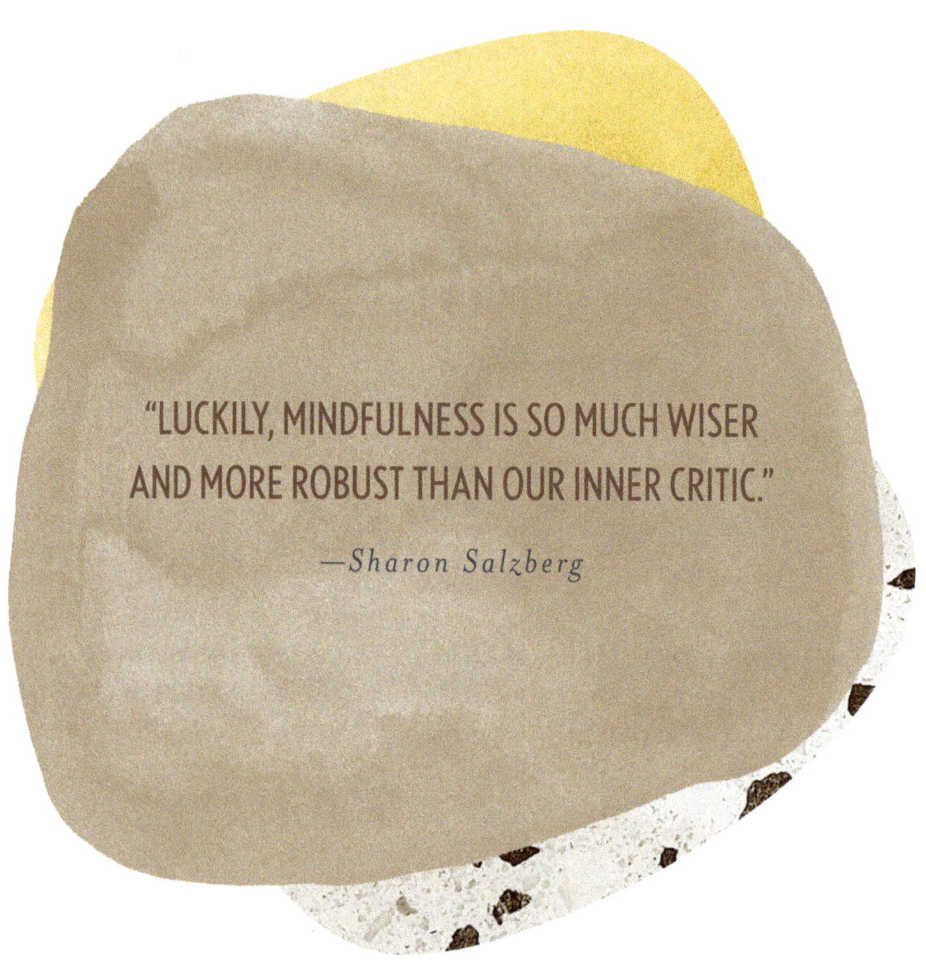

"LUCKILY, MINDFULNESS IS SO MUCH WISER AND MORE ROBUST THAN OUR INNER CRITIC."

—Sharon Salzberg

DEPRESSION CAN MAKE it difficult to eat in nourishing ways, yet when you eat the right amount and type of food, you give your brain and body the fuel it needs to stay clear and uncluttered for optimal performance. List some simple, healthy foods that you have enjoyed eating.

SELECT ONE OF your favorite foods from the list. Close your eyes and imagine yourself eating it. Describe in detail how the food looks, smells, feels (in your hands and in your mouth), and tastes.

MINDFUL MOVEMENT: CAT-COW STRETCH

This gentle yoga stretch loosens muscles, stimulates energy flow through the spine and entire nervous system, and helps you connect your breath to your body's motion. Do this any time you notice tightness in your body or are feeling tired and sluggish.

- Begin on the floor on all fours. Alternatively, sit on the edge of a chair, or position yourself in any way that is comfortable for you.
- As you inhale slowly and deeply, tilt your head and hips to the sky while letting your belly dip down toward the floor. (It won't come close to touching the floor.)
- As you exhale, gradually round your back and let your head and hips drop toward the floor.
- Repeat, breathing slowly in and out as you dip and round your spine.

DESCRIBE SOMETHING NICE someone has done for you; something that makes you feel loved and grateful.

DESCRIBE SOMETHING KIND you have done for someone to make their day a little brighter.

WHAT ARE YOU curious or intrigued about beyond the boundaries of your depression? List people, places, animals, objects, topics, or ideas you'd like to know more about.

MAKE A POINT to experience each moment fully by dedicating time, one moment at a time, to nurturing your curiosity. Circle two things you will do this week to learn more about one topic or idea you just listed. Write down the days you will explore.

I will broaden my horizons and follow my curiosity by . . .

- Searching for online articles and reading one
- Browsing through catalogs and magazines to find related images and creating a collage
- Visiting my library and wandering through the related section to find one book to check out
- Watching one video about the topic
- Downloading an app dedicated to the idea and spending 5 to 10 minutes exploring it
- Asking someone I know to share their knowledge with me
- Finding "how-to" instructions to make something on my own
-
-
-
-

THE WAITING GAME

Waiting (in long lines, at red lights, for water to boil, etc.) can be annoying, and it gives your mind the opportunity to wander, sometimes to places you don't want it to go. Turn these intrusive "downtimes" into mindful moments and nurture your mood. Use these opportunities to breathe and notice your thoughts and feelings. Then, expand your awareness to the things around you, concentrating on random sights, sounds, scents, and textures. You can even make the waiting game playful by challenging yourself to spot as many red items as you can, or trying to identify four different sounds before the waiting period ends.

IT'S TIME TO pause to appreciate your progress! Look back through part 2. You spent time noticing unpleasant thoughts, feelings, and experiences, yet you stuck with it even if it may have been difficult. Write a letter of appreciation to yourself for hanging in there. Remind yourself of the strength and courage you had to muster.

WHAT DOES "LIVING a life of meaning" mean to you? For some, this means spending quality time with family. For others, it means traveling or engaging in a specific type of activity. The answer is personal, and as long as it doesn't bring harm to yourself or others, there are no wrong answers.

ON A SCALE from 1 to 10, with 1 representing "not at all" and 10 representing "completely," how meaningful does your life feel to you?

not at all — 1 2 3 4 5 6 7 8 9 10 — *completely*

Describe people, places, and/or activities that already create a sense of meaning.

HOW CAN YOU move yourself up the scale by a single number? Brainstorm a go-to list of things you could do, one day or one moment at a time, to deepen your sense of purpose. (You might slip people short, positive notes, help someone with a task, use your skills to make something for someone, etc.)

OCEAN BREATH

This mindful breathing exercise evokes the sound and imagery of ocean waves rhythmically ebbing and flowing.

- Sit or lie comfortably. Ensure that your spine is straight and shoulders are relaxed.
- Close your eyes or lower your gaze.
- Place the tip of your tongue softly against the roof of your mouth just behind your front teeth. Slightly constrict your throat as if you were going to whisper.
- Inhale slowly through your nose. Listen to the sound the air makes as it moves down into your lungs.
- Exhale slowly through your mouth, again being attentive to the sound.
- As you breathe, imagine ocean waves lapping and receding.

DEPRESSION RESTRICTS YOUR perspective so you automatically focus on negative aspects of people or situations. Think of someone or something that is difficult, and broaden your perspective. Without denying anything troublesome, zoom out your mental picture a bit wider and describe other characteristics of the person or other things that are happening in addition to the difficult situation.

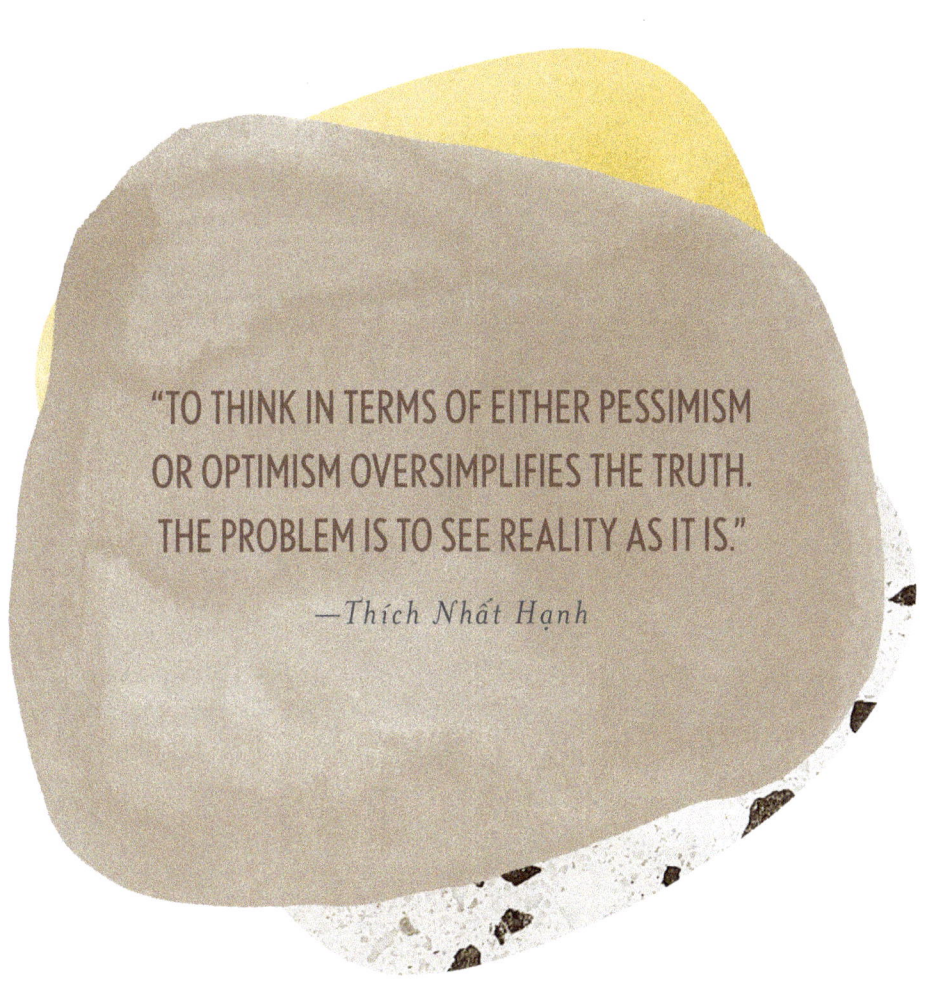

"TO THINK IN TERMS OF EITHER PESSIMISM OR OPTIMISM OVERSIMPLIFIES THE TRUTH. THE PROBLEM IS TO SEE REALITY AS IT IS."

—*Thích Nhất Hạnh*

WHEN YOU'RE STUCK in the negative thoughts and experiences of depression, you sometimes miss out on pleasurable experiences. Practice savoring positive moments. Close your eyes and recall something or someone that has brought you joy. Describe this event or person fully here, using details from your senses.

CREATE A PLAYLIST of uplifting or inspiring songs or other sounds to listen to in a moment of low mood. Here, begin a list of some of your all-time favorite songs, genres, or artists. You can also include nature sounds, meditation bells, or chanting tracks. What lifts you the moment you start to hear it?

RIGHT NOW, WHAT is your depression telling you about yourself, another person, or a situation in your life? What emotions are you feeling? How is this affecting what you feel like doing (or not doing)?

SELECT ONE OF the songs you listed on page 161, and play it now. (You might be able to find a lyric video on YouTube or search for the song on a music service app such as Spotify or Pandora.) Immerse yourself in the music mindfully. Feel your body respond to the beat and pay attention to the words. Appreciate the talent of the performers. When the experience has ended, write about the thoughts and emotions you are now experiencing. How has your motivation changed?

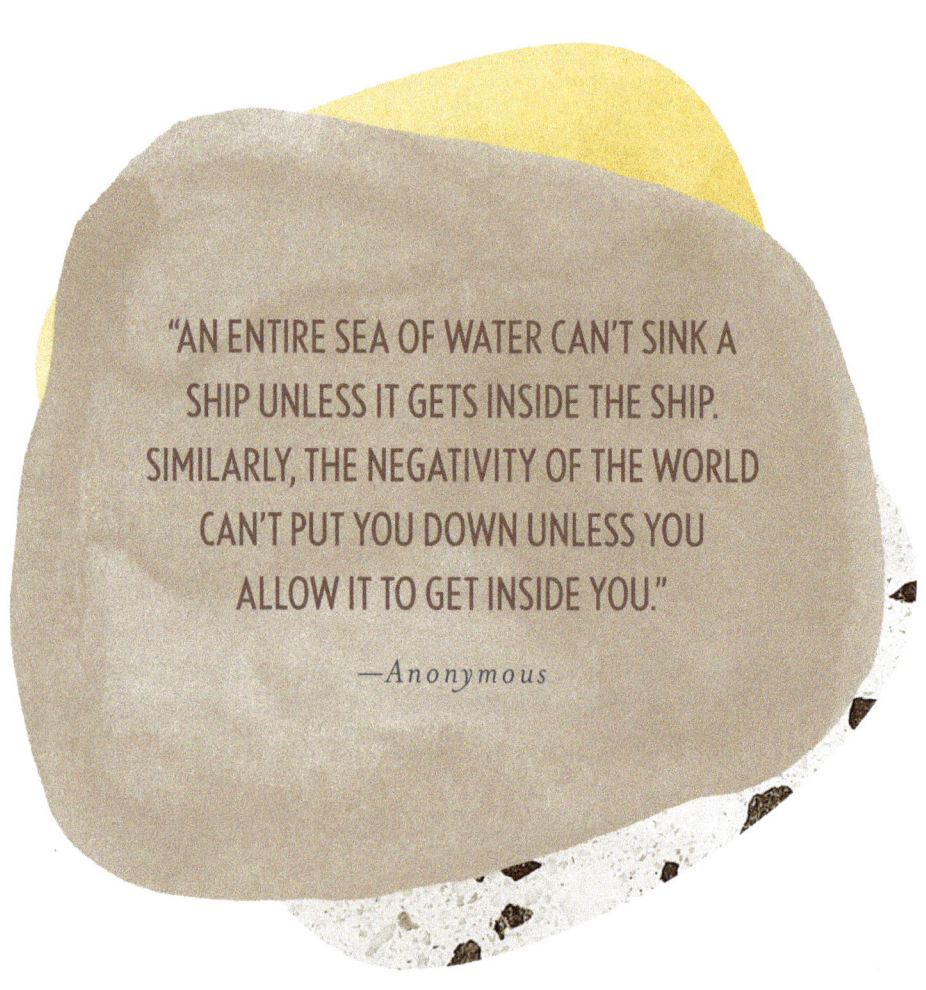

"AN ENTIRE SEA OF WATER CAN'T SINK A SHIP UNLESS IT GETS INSIDE THE SHIP. SIMILARLY, THE NEGATIVITY OF THE WORLD CAN'T PUT YOU DOWN UNLESS YOU ALLOW IT TO GET INSIDE YOU."

—*Anonymous*

MINDFUL TASKS

Every moment is a chance to be mindfully engaged in life. As you go about each day, break the habit of operating on autopilot while your mind runs away with your mood. When you are doing the dishes, cleaning a surface, or doing the laundry, for example, attend to the task as if it were the most important thing in the world. (After all, it *is* important because it is what you are doing in that moment, the only moment that tangibly exists.) Note and savor sensory details. When you are with others, enjoy the experience by paying complete attention to these people who are part of your moment.

LEARNING TO BE mindful is like building a muscle. To help you "train," return to this list of mindfulness characteristics every day and put a big star, heart, or other symbol on an item to indicate that you've sought and found something positive. Reflect below on how those positive moments have helped shift your day (even incrementally!)

- Pulling my thoughts out of my mind and into a moment
- Spending time with a loved one
- Unexpected downtime
- Doing a task despite difficulties
- Catching my inner critic and shifting my thoughts to one of my strengths
- Expressing my love to someone
- Exploring my curiosity
- Listening to music
- Feeling proud of a personal trait
- Acknowledging when something went well
- Receiving a positive comment
- Doing a small act of kindness for a stranger
- Receiving a small act of kindness from a stranger
- Laughing
- Identifying a positive person in my life
- Stopping and smelling the roses
- Visualizing a fond memory
- Being with someone who fully listens to me
- Looking at a cherished photo and smiling
- Remembering something that made me happy today
- Hearing someone laugh
- Spending time in nature
- Getting lost in a good book
- Creating something

TREAT YOURSELF WITH lovingkindness, a well-known attitude and approach of gentle compassion, understanding, and forgiveness. A standard lovingkindness meditation involves closing your eyes, breathing slowly and deeply, and gently telling yourself, "May I be safe. May I be healthy. May I be happy. May I live with ease." Go deep with this. What does safety mean to you? Health? Happiness? Ease of being? How will you fill your life with these qualities?

CELEBRATE!

You have so much to celebrate. You have many strengths. You're taking charge of your life by embracing a mindful way of living and expanding your focus. As you grow, you're breaking down the walls of depression. Purposefully celebrate this, and celebrate yourself. Small celebrations, such as a little happy dance or raising your teacup and saying "Cheers!" boost confidence and reinforce the pleasure pathways in your brain. Even tiny celebrations pave the way for more success, and they help you feel pleasure. Cheers to you and your progress!

YOU'VE MADE IT! Look back to the very first response you made in this journal (page 2). You reflected on the thoughts, experiences, and feelings that prompted you to pick up this book. What has changed since then? How is your relationship with those thoughts, experiences, and feelings different? Celebrate your growth by doing something nice for yourself, and experiencing it mindfully!

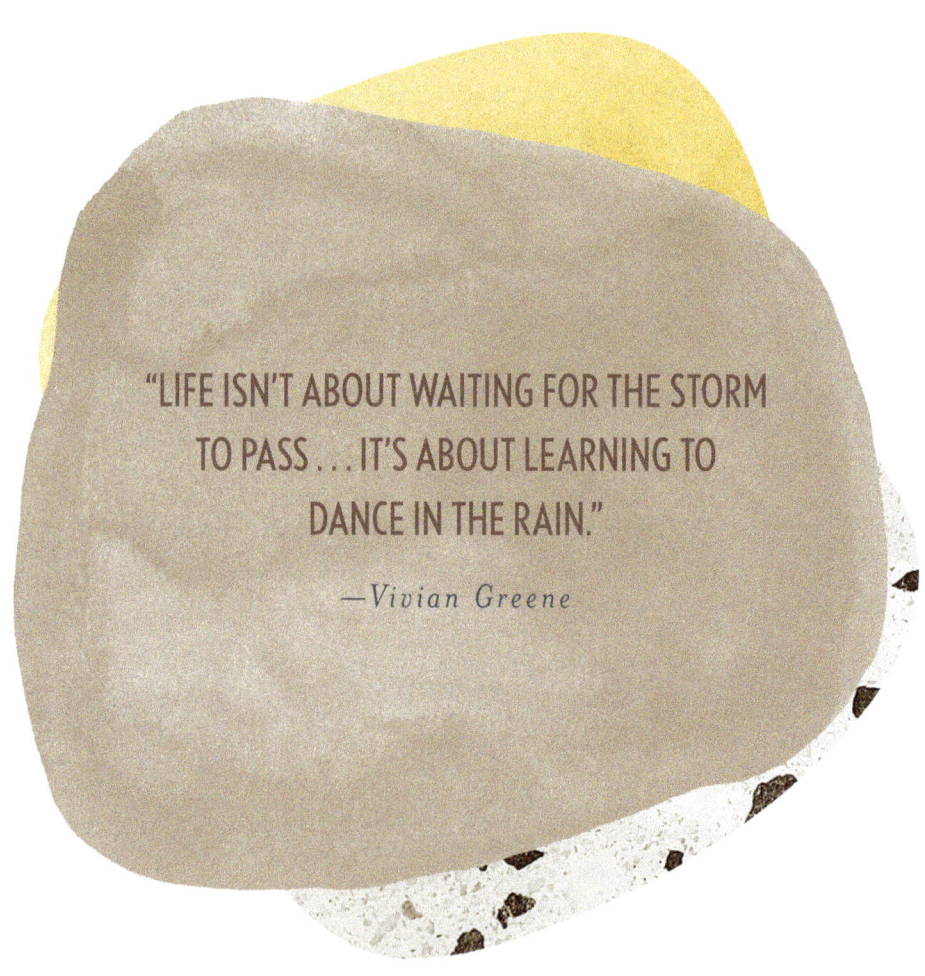

"LIFE ISN'T ABOUT WAITING FOR THE STORM TO PASS... IT'S ABOUT LEARNING TO DANCE IN THE RAIN."

—*Vivian Greene*

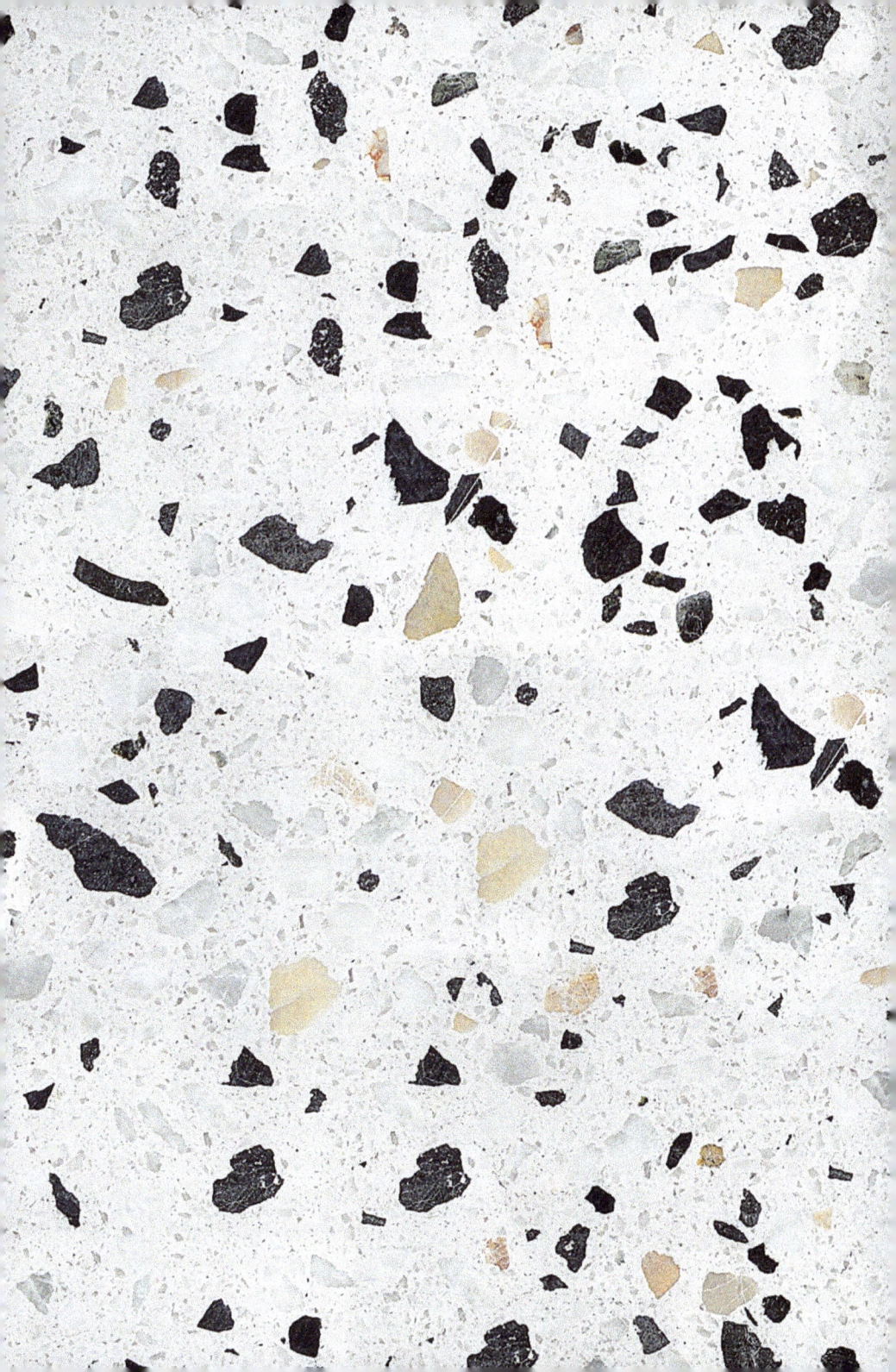

RESOURCES

To learn more about overcoming depression through mindfulness, check out these sources:

Books

Mindfulness for Beginners: Reclaiming the Present Moment—and Your Life, by Jon Kabat-Zinn. This book offers insights and practical exercises to help you embrace mindfulness as a way of life.

The Mindfulness Workbook for Depression: Effective Mindfulness Strategies to Cultivate Positivity from the Inside Out, by Yoon Im Kane. Use mindfulness strategies to explore negative thought patterns and work past depression symptoms that are holding you back from your life.

Peace Is Every Step: The Path of Mindfulness in Everyday Life, by Thích Nhất Hạnh. Harness the power of mindfulness by reading brief stories, personal examples, and short, practical exercises.

Websites

Depression and Bipolar Support Alliance (DBSA). Learn about depression and find resources for support online or at a local DBSA office. DBSAlliance.org

HelpGuide.org. This health and wellness organization offers a useful article on how to exercise with limited ability. HelpGuide.org/articles/healthy-living/chair-exercises-and-limited-mobility-fitness.htm

MBCT.com. This is the online home of mindfulness-based cognitive therapy (MBCT). Learn detailed information about MBCT and where to find group classes if interested. MBCT.com

National Alliance on Mental Illness (NAMI). Discover information, resources, and support for depression. Find information online or at a NAMI affiliate center near you. NAMI.org

The Free Mindfulness Project. An online resource providing information about mindfulness as well as numerous free, downloadable mindfulness exercises. FreeMindfulness.org

UCSD Center for Mindfulness. Housed within the University of California San Diego School of Medicine, the Center for Mindfulness offers a wealth of information and optional online courses about using mindfulness in everyday life. MedSchool.ucsd.edu/som/fmph/research/mindfulness/Pages/default.aspx

VIA Character. An outstanding resource for scientifically valid information about universal character strengths. You can take a free assessment of your unique strengths and learn more about strengths and how to use them. VIACharacter.org

Online Courses

Be Mindful Online Mindfulness Course. This online, self-paced course helps you learn and develop mindfulness skills to reduce depression, stress, anxiety, and other challenges. BeMindfulOnline.com

Centre for Mindfulness Studies Online MBCT Program. Participate in a live, online MBCT program from the Toronto, Canada-based organization for mindfulness-based mental health interventions. MindfulnessStudies.com/personal/mbct-online

UMass Memorial Medical Center MBCT Online. Take an online MBCT course from the place where mindfulness-based group programs first originated. UMMHealth.org/umass-memorial-medical-center/services-treatments/center-for-mindfulness/mindfulness-programs/mbct-8-week-online-live

Helplines

If you feel overwhelmed and in crisis, know that you are not alone. Feeling this way is so universal that many helplines exist to assist. They lend listening ears, and they can point you to helpful, supportive resources in your community. These are some of the prominent helplines that are available 24/7.

National Suicide Prevention Lifeline: Designed for people of all ages and backgrounds, this helpline is accessible via phone or online chat. 1-800-273-TALK (8255) or SuicidePreventionLifeline.org

SAMHSA's National Helpline: The Substance Abuse and Mental Health Services Administration offers this helpline for anyone experiencing a crisis due to substance use or mental health disorders, including depression. 1-800-662-HELP (4357)

Crisis Text Line: This service offers help for anyone experiencing depression. Text HOME to 741741 for instant connection to a crisis counselor.

The Trevor Project: A national helpline service for LGBTQIA+ youth, the Trevor Project has phone, online chat, and texting crisis support. Call 1-866-488-7386, Text START to 678-678, or go to TheTrevorProject.org/get-help-now/ to chat online.

Trans Lifeline: This group provides support to the trans community from the trans community. 1-877-565-8860

REFERENCES

Beck, Aaron T. "Negative Core Beliefs in CBT." Beck Institute for Cognitive Behavior Therapy. January 8, 2014. BeckInstitute.org/negative-core-beliefs-in-cbt.

Burns, David D. *The Feeling Good Handbook*. New York: Plume, 1999.

Campbell, Polly. "Why You Should Celebrate Everything." *Psychology Today*. December 2, 2015. PsychologyToday.com/us/blog/imperfect-spirituality/201512/why-you-should-celebrate-everything.

Chödrön, Pema. "Don't Bite the Hook." *Tricycle Magazine*. Summer 2009. Tricycle.org/magazine/dont-bite-hook.

———. "How We Get Hooked and How We Get Unhooked." *Lion's Roar*. December 26, 2017. LionsRoar.com/how-we-get-hooked-shenpa-and-how-we-get-unhooked.

Colier, Nancy. "Why Your Thoughts Are Not Real." *Psychology Today*. August 23, 2013. PsychologyToday.com/us/blog/inviting-monkey-tea/201308/why-your-thoughts-are-not-real.

Gibran, Kahlil. *Sand and Foam: A Book of Aphorisms*. New York: Alfred A. Knopf, 2001.

Gillihan, Seth J. "7 Ways Yoga Lowers Stress and Anxiety." *Psychology Today*. September 15, 2016. PsychologyToday.com/us/blog/think-act-be/201609/7-ways-yoga-lowers-stress-and-anxiety.

Goldstein, Elisha. "Thoughts Are Not Facts." *Mindful*. January 7, 2016. Mindful.org/thoughts-are-not-facts.

Hạnh, Thích Nhất. *Peace Is Every Step: The Path of Mindfulness in Everyday Life*. New York: Bantam, 1992.

Harvard Men's Health Watch. "Sour Mood Getting You Down? Get Back to Nature." *Harvard Health Publishing: Harvard Medical School*. March 30, 2021. Health.Harvard.edu/mind-and-mood/sour-mood-getting-you-down-get-back-to-nature.

Harvard Mental Health Letter. "Yoga Can Blunt Harmful Effects of Stress, from the Harvard Mental Health Letter." *Harvard Health Publishing: Harvard Medical School*. April 1, 2009. Health.Harvard.edu/press_releases/yoga-can-blunt-harmful-effects-of-stress.

Hofmann, Stefan G., Alice T. Sawyer, Ashley A. Witt, and Diana Oh. "The Effect of Mindfulness-Based Therapy on Anxiety and Depression: A Meta-Analytic Review." *Journal of Consulting and Clinical Psychology* 78, no. 2 (April 2010): 169–83. DOI.org/10.1037/a0018555.

Jerath, Ravinder, John W. Edry, Vernon A. Barnes, and Vandna Jerath. "Physiology of Long Pranayamic Breathing: Neural Respiratory Elements May Provide a Mechanism That Explains How Slow Deep Breathing Shifts the Autonomic Nervous System." *Medical Hypotheses* 67, no. 3 (February 2006): 566–71. DOI.org/10.1016/j.mehy.2006.02.042.

Kabat-Zinn, Jon. *Coming to Our Senses: Healing Ourselves and the World Through Mindfulness*. New York: Hachette Books, 2005.

———. *Full Catastrophe Living: Using the Wisdom of Your Body and Mind to Face Stress, Pain, and Illness*. Revised ed. New York: Bantam, 2013.

———. *Mindfulness for Beginners: Reclaiming the Present Moment and Your Life*. Boulder, CO: Sounds True, 2016.

Mayo Clinic Staff. "Yoga: Fight Stress and Find Serenity." *Mayo Clinic Healthy Lifestyle*. December 29, 2020. MayoClinic.org/healthy-lifestyle/stress-management/in-depth/yoga/art-20044733.

MBCT.com. "How Does Mindfulness Help Reduce Downward Mood Spirals?" Accessed April 2021. MBCT.com/how-does-mindfulness-help-reduce-downward-mood-spirals.html.

———. "Welcome to MBCT.com." Accessed April 2021. MBCT.com.

Mind.org. "Nature and Mental Health: How Can I Overcome Barriers?" May 2018. Mind.org.uk/information-support/tips-for-everyday-living/nature-and-mental-health/overcoming-barriers.

Niemiec, Ryan M. *Mindfulness & Character Strengths: A Practical Guide to Flourishing*. Boston: Hogrefe, 2014.

Peterson, Tanya J. "Mindfulness-Based Cognitive Therapy: How It Works, Cost, & What to Expect." *Choosing Therapy*. Last modified February 23, 2021. ChoosingTherapy.com/mindfulness-based-cognitive-therapy.

Psychology Today Staff. "Mindfulness-Based Cognitive Therapy." *Psychology Today*. Accessed April 2021. PsychologyToday.com/us/therapy-types/mindfulness-based-cognitive-therapy.

Raghunathan, Raj. "How Negative Is Your 'Mental Chatter'?" *Psychology Today*. October 10, 2013. PsychologyToday.com/us/blog/sapient-nature/201310/how-negative-is-your-mental-chatter.

Ray, Amit. *Mindfulness: Living in the Moment—Living in the Breath*. Atlanta, GA: Inner Light Publishers, 2015.

Rivera, Angel. "Everything You Need to Know About Mindfulness-Based Cognitive Therapy (MBCT)." *Depression Alliance*. Accessed on April 2021. DepressionAlliance.org/mindfulness-based-cognitive-therapy.

Robbins, Jim. "Ecopsychology: How Immersion in Nature Benefits Your Health." *Yale Environment 360*. January 9, 2020. e360.Yale.edu/features/ecopsychology-how-immersion-in-nature-benefits-your-health.

Salzberg, Sharon. *Real Love: The Art of Mindful Connection*. New York: Flatiron Books, 2017.

Segerstrom, Suzanne. "The Structure and Consequences of Repetitive Thought." *Psychological Science Agenda*. March 2011. APA.org/science/about/psa/2011/03/repetitive-thought.

Sipe, Walter E. B., and Stuart J. Eisendrath. "Mindfulness-Based Cognitive Therapy: Theory and Practice." *The Canadian Journal of Psychiatry* 57, no. 2 (February 2012): 63–69. DOI.org/10.1177/070674371205700202.

Streeter, Chris, et al. "Effects of Yoga Versus Walking on Mood, Anxiety, and Brain GABA Levels: A Randomized Controlled MRS Study." *The Journal of Alternative and Complementary Medicine* 16, no. 11 (November 2010):1145–52. DOI.org/10.1089/acm.2010.0007.

TEDx Talks. "The Mindful Way through Depression: Zindel Segal at TEDxUTSC." YouTube Video, 18:04. April 22, 2014. YouTube.com/watch?v=1A4w3W94ygA.

Trungpa, Chögyam. *Mindfulness in Action: Making Friends with Yourself through Meditation and Everyday Awareness*. Boulder, CO: Shambhala Publications, 2016.

VIA Institute on Character. "Character Strengths." Accessed May 2021. VIACharacter.org/character-strengths-via.

White, Mathew P., et al. "Spending at Least 120 Minutes a Week in Nature Is Associated with Good Health and Well-being." *Scientific Reports* 9, no. 3 (June 2019): 7730. Nature.com/articles/s41598-019-44097-3.

Acknowledgments

I am deeply grateful for the guidance and assistance offered by the talented team at Callisto Media. Thank you for believing in me. Thank you, too, for providing feedback and lending your insights to help make the *Mindfulness Journal for Depression* a strong, reliable, and useful tool for helping people form a new relationship with themselves and their lives and embrace each moment fully, exactly as it is.

About the Author

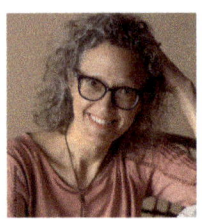

Tanya J. Peterson holds a Master of Science degree in counseling, is credentialed by the National Board of Certified Counselors, and is a Diplomate of the American Institute of Stress. She is the author of eight self-help books and a regular contributor to a variety of mental health websites. Formerly a teacher and school counselor, Peterson has also created a mental health course to help kids develop the skills needed to deal positively with worries, stress, and other problems. She's been a guest on numerous podcasts and other interview shows, such as the *Empowered Living* talk show on Facebook, the American Institute of Stress's *Finding Contentment* podcast, and many more. She has a webinar offered through the American Institute of Stress. Peterson has been featured twice in *Authority Magazine* regarding developing healthy habits for well-being and leveraging the power of gratitude for wellness. She's been quoted as an expert in a variety of online articles on WebMD and Verywell Mind. Her work centers on helping people understand and build mindfulness skills in order to live fully in each moment rather than stuck in their thoughts and feelings about problematic situations.

www.ingramcontent.com/pod-product-compliance
Lightning Source LLC
LaVergne TN
LVHW010305070426
835507LV00027B/3443